Synthesizing qualitative and quantitative health evidence

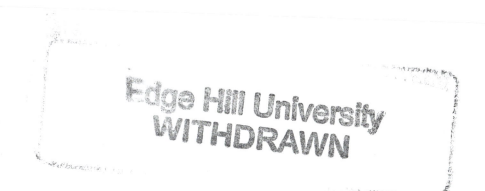

Synthesizing qualitative and quantitative health evidence

A guide to methods

*Catherine Pope, Nicholas Mays and
Jennie Popay*

 Open University Press

Open University Press
McGraw-Hill Education
McGraw-Hill House
Shoppenhangers Road
Maidenhead
Berkshire
England
SL6 2QL

email: enquiries@openup.co.uk
world wide web: www.openup.co.uk

and Two Penn Plaza, New York, NY 10121-2289, USA

First published 2007

A catalogue record of this book is available from the British Library

ISBN-13: 978 0 335 21956 8 (pb) 978 0 335 21957 5 (hb)
ISBN-10: 0 335 21956 X (pb) 0 335 21957 8 (hb)

Library of Congress Cataloging-in-Publication Data
CIP data applied for

Typeset by RefineCatch Limited, Bungay, Suffolk
Printed in Poland by OZGraf S.A.
www.polskabook.pl

The *McGraw·Hill* Companies

Contents

About the authors   vi

Preface   vii

Acknowledgements   x

PART 1
The evidence review process   1

1 Different types of evidence review   3
2 Stages in reviewing evidence systematically   19

PART 2
Methods for evidence synthesis   45

3 Quantitative approaches to evidence synthesis   47
4 Interpretive approaches to evidence synthesis   72
5 Mixed approaches to evidence synthesis   95

PART 3
The product of evidence synthesis   115

6 Organising and presenting evidence synthesis   117
7 Using evidence reviews for policy- and decision-making   153
8 Approaches and assessment: choosing different methods and considering quality   171

Useful reading   187

References   191

Index   205

About the authors

Catherine Pope and Nicholas Mays previously edited the highly successful *Qualitative Research in Health Care* (3rd edition 2006, Blackwell Publishing) and Nicholas and Jennie Popay collaborated in writing the chapter on synthesizing research evidence in the methods textbook *Studying the Organisation and Delivery of Health Services* (2001, Routledge). Jennie also edited *Moving Beyond Effectiveness in Evidence Synthesis: Methodological Issues in the Synthesis of Diverse Sources of Evidence* published in 2006 by the UK National Institute for Health and Clinical Excellence (NICE). Catherine is Reader in Health Services Research at the University of Southampton. She has been involved in developing methods for the synthesis of qualitative methods and undertakes primary research on health care organisation and innovation, and professional practice. Nicholas is a part-time health policy advisor to the New Zealand Treasury where he is a doer, user and commissioner of reviews, and he combines this with the role of Professor of Health Policy at the London School of Hygiene and Tropical Medicine. Jennie is Professor of Sociology and Public Health at the Institute for Health Research at the University of Lancaster. She has played an active part in encouraging the health research communities to include qualitative research within the ambit of systematic reviews of the effectiveness of health care and established the Cochrane Qualitative Research Methods Group (which she now jointly convenes) and the Campbell Implementation Methods Group.

Preface

This book is a guide to how to synthesize diverse sources of evidence so that they are most likely to be useful for policy and managerial decision-making. It was written with those working as researchers, policy-makers or practitioners in the field of health in mind, but will be of use to those working in other areas of social and public policy such as education, welfare, crime and prisons, housing and so on. It is aimed at researchers (rather than decision-makers themselves) who want to conduct reviews to inform decision-making but recognise that the questions decision-makers ask are complex – for example, questions that go beyond 'what works?' and ask in addition 'when?' 'how?' and 'why?' as well as 'for which people in which circumstances?' Often the answers to these questions are located in a variety of research and non-research sources, and some of the answers may come from unpublished as well as published materials. Synthesis offers a way of understanding and using these diverse sources of evidence. Many of the methods discussed in this book have been designed to synthesize published qualitative and quantitative research findings, but some could, potentially at least, be extended to synthesize other kinds of evidence. This book describes how to undertake a review but its central focus is evidence synthesis – that part of the review process which seeks to combine and integrate evidence.

Much of what has found its way into this book developed from an overview of methods for synthesizing qualitative and quantitative evidence (Mays et al. 2005). In addition to this work, each us has also undertaken primary research on issues linked to policy on public health and health services. Engagement with this type of research almost inevitably brings researchers into contact with a range of decision-makers, including national policy-makers, commissioners of research, and local managers and practitioners who are looking for answers to questions about health care services and delivery, and ways of improving population health and reducing health inequalities. This book details some of the methods we have found for bridging the so-called 'gap' between evidence and policy which should make reviews more useful to these decision-makers. Many of the examples used in the book are drawn from health – principally because this is the field we know best – but we hope that the book will be equally useful to researchers and reviewers of evidence in other fields of applied social research.

As well as being applied researchers we are all also practitioners of what are called 'mixed methods' approaches to research and evaluation. We are familiar with qualitative and quantitative approaches to research but it is probably fair to note that we have each, at various points, championed qualitative approaches against the traditional dominance of quantitative approaches in medicine, health services and public health research (Pope and Mays 1993; Popay and Williams 1998). In many ways we see evidence synthesis as a natural extension of this mixed approach and we are very interested in broadening the scope of what 'counts' as evidence in the kinds of review and report which are designed to inform decision-making. For us, evidence includes quantitative and qualitative research findings, as well as other forms of evidence such as stakeholder surveys or the views and values of experts and users. In our view the inclusion of diverse sources of evidence in reviews does not mean abandoning the rigour of systematic reviews, but it does mean judging the quality of evidence in context and defining evidence as relevant to answering specific questions, rather than defining some forms of evidence as intrinsically, and universally, of lower quality than others.

Why do we need evidence synthesis? Despite, or perhaps because of, the growth in the evidence available (which is described in Chapter 1) there has been a failure to build a cumulative evidence base in many areas of health policy. For researchers designing research this means it is difficult to identify the gaps and the new questions that need answering, and it may mean that research time is spent retracing the ground covered by previous studies. The lack of cumulation is also a problem for funders and commissioners of research in deciding where to target their limited resources. Synthesis may help to map out the terrain for all these players. Another major strength of synthesis is its potential contribution to policy- and decision-making in fields such as health care where it might allow us to integrate and make connections between qualitative and quantitative research findings.

Outline of the book

The book is divided into three parts. The first part looks in detail at reviewing evidence. Chapter 1 looks at the development of different types of review, and the emergence of systematic reviewing. It examines the rationale for conducting synthesis and the distinction between reviews for 'decision support' and for 'knowledge support'. Chapter 2 takes a more detailed look at the stages entailed in reviewing evidence systematically and includes a discussion of the issues surrounding quality appraisal of research evidence.

Part 2 focuses on different approaches to evidence synthesis which are potentially useful when the body of evidence includes qualitative and quantitative research findings. One simple way of differentiating between approaches is to distinguish between those that are broadly quantitative (i.e. methods that involve numbers and statistical analysis) and those which are more qualitative or text-based. Indeed this is an approach we have taken in the past (Mays et al. 2005). However, in writing this book we have found it more helpful to delineate three types of approach to synthesis: those that deal with numerical data; those which typically deal with qualitative data but which are linked by an interpretive focus; and finally a broader category which, for want of a better term, we have called 'mixed' approaches to synthesis. These may include qualitative and/or quantitative analytical methods as part of a review process. With this typology in mind, Chapter 3 describes a number of approaches to synthesis which allow the statistical analysis or numerically-based logical (Boolean) analysis. Chapter 4 outlines approaches to synthesis which are broadly qualitative and interpretative in nature. The final chapter of Part 2, Chapter 5, broadens out the focus to examine a variety of approaches to evidence synthesis which do not readily align with the quantitative or interpretive approaches to synthesis and are best described as 'mixed' approaches to synthesis. These approaches include narrative forms that can incorporate one or several of the methods already described.

Part 3 focuses on the product of synthesis. Chapter 6 explores different ways of presenting the findings of an evidence synthesis, focusing particularly on synthesis as part of a systematic review. This includes consideration of how to be transparent about the process of synthesis in order to reveal an audit trail that readers can scrutinise. Chapter 7 looks at the place of synthesis in reviews for policy and management. It looks at the role of evidence in decision-making and considers why different sorts of evidence are ignored and whether there are ways of 'doing' synthesis that overcome these limitations. Chapter 8 provides an overview and concluding points about the process of conducting and interpreting a synthesis of qualitative–quantitative evidence. In particular it explores the choice of appropriate techniques to answer different types of question and to handle different types of evidence. Finally it presents a list of questions which can be used to assess the quality of a synthesis of diverse evidence.

Acknowledgements

The overview of methods for synthesizing qualitative and quantitative evidence (Mays et al. 2005) was commissioned and funded by the Canadian Health Services Research Foundation (CHSRF) and the English NHS Service Delivery Organisation (SDO) R and D Programme. Alongside this work we participated in a series of meetings which brought together methodologists, policy-makers, researchers and funders all grappling with the problem of how to inform and support decision-making by managers, practitioners and policy-makers in the health care sector. Conversations and debates about synthesis with these experts made a significant contribution to our thinking about methods for synthesis and we acknowledge our debt of gratitude to all the participants in this evidence synthesis endeavour. In addition to the above review, Jennie Popay has been involved in the preparation of guidance in the conduct of narrative synthesis in systematic reviews funded by the UK Economic and Social Research Council (Popay et al. forthcoming). This guidance, which is described in Chapter 5, has also made an important contribution to our understanding of the issues and debates surrounding the development of review methodology and we would therefore like to thank the rest of the team of researchers involved in this project: Helen Roberts, Amanda Sowden, Mark Petticrew, Lisa Arai, Mark Rodgers, Nicky Britten, Katrina Roen and Steven Duffy. Sally Baldwin, also a valued member of this team, died as a result of an accident during the project.

PART 1
The evidence review process

1 Different types of evidence review

Every year a vast number of health-related research studies are carried out. There are randomised controlled trials of new treatments, surveys of patient experiences, evaluations of interventions designed to improve health and/or reduce health inequalities, analyses of routinely collected hospital episode statistics, economic evaluations of the costs and effectiveness of health care, case studies of new practice, research on the experience of service users, patients and health care professionals and so on. This research is conducted by researchers from a diverse range of disciplinary and professional backgrounds, including statistics, epidemiology, psychology, sociology, anthropology, political and economic science, geography, public health and the medical, nursing and therapy professions, and it draws on a variety of different theoretical and methodological approaches. As a result of all this research activity, each week journal papers, books and reports add to the already vast number of publications about the effects and impacts of health interventions, the experience of illness and health care, and the organisation and reorganisation of health-related services. These studies are published in social science, medical, nursing and health-related journals, in books and monographs, and increasingly as electronic publications, online. Alongside this published literature there is also a large but less visible 'grey' or unpublished literature which includes research reports, policy briefings and unpublished dissertations. There are also other types of evidence which might inform policy- and decision-making such as consultations with expert and lay groups, and a host of different types of information available via the World Wide Web.

There is growing awareness of the need to strengthen the link between knowledge derived from this mountain of diverse evidence and the decisions made in health care policy and practice (Haines et al. 2004). Surely all this evidence can tell us what should be prioritised, funded, and developed? Unfortunately there are problems with relying on this evidence. Some studies may be too small to provide reliable and valid evidence. Other evidence may be context-bound – specific to a particular country, a region or much smaller unit of analysis such as a group of patients – such that it is difficult to see which findings are most salient and/or how the findings might be applied in another context. Some research is biased by flaws in the study design or methods, and this makes using the findings highly problematic. Research may tackle only one small part of the question or problem which decision-makers want to know about: unpublished studies and other sources of evidence need to be drawn on. There are often additional problems with determining the quality and rigour of non-research sources of evidence.

This information mountain, and the methodological and other problems associated with it, presents major challenges for policy-makers, managers and practitioners (Petticrew and Roberts 2006: 7). The sheer volume of evidence increases daily as more research reports are published adding to the volumes of journals and books, and these are joined by different types of unpublished and non-research material. The expansion of information technologies, notably the World Wide Web, has exacerbated this information overload rather than controlling it. Web-based sources of information about research allow access to more evidence, but with the additional problem of uncertainty as to the relevance, reliability and quality of material from such sources.

Dealing with the information mountain – reviewing the evidence

First generation 'traditional' literature reviews

Literature reviews are a well-established method in the social sciences for trying to bring together evidence from research. These reviews have been referred to as narrative reviews (Dixon-Woods et al. 2004; Pawson and Bellaby 2006) although this label can be confusing as some narrative approaches to synthesis are far more methodologically rigorous than traditional literature reviews and can form part of systematic review processes. In the past, literature reviews were typically conducted by acknowledged 'experts' in the field, who would collect together individual studies they were familiar with, and attempt to make sense of the cumulative evidence by summarising and interpreting that literature. A literature review remains an essential precursor to research, a way of locating where previous research has reached, identifying the gaps and where to look next. This approach to literature reviewing still forms the basis of most doctoral theses and is often the format for the opening chapter of research reports. Many reviews written in this way make excellent reading and may well be regarded as providing sufficient of an overview to inform future research and decision-making.

However, what might be termed 'first generation' or traditional literature reviews paid little, if any, attention to assessing the methodological quality of the studies included or to searching systematically for all potentially relevant evidence. Rather they tended to focus on selectively gathering and reviewing evidence that provided both context and substance to the authors' overall arguments. Authors could be highly subjective, biased or plain ignorant in their choice of literature and interpretation. Few were critical of the research they included, and poorly designed and executed studies might be reviewed alongside high quality ones with little consideration given to how study quality might affect the results and the weight to be given to different sources of evidence. First generation reviews have been rightly criticised for a lack of transparency in the methods adopted for gathering and reviewing literature and for a lack of attention to the important issue of bias. However, as the review of research on anti-social behaviour by Rutter and colleagues (1998) illustrates (Box 1.1) it would be a mistake to assume that all such literature reviews necessarily lack sophistication in the review process or that they cannot contribute to the production of new knowledge or theory.

Box 1.1 A critical appraisal of a first generation literature review: research on anti-social behaviour (Rutter et al. 1998)

1. Telling a convincing story
The authorial voice is central to the power of this literature review helping to draw the reader through a complex array of material, painting a clear and coherent picture of the literature being reviewed and establishing a tone of authority and trustworthiness. The authors have essentially selected studies to provide both context for and substance to the story they are developing.

2. Developing a theoretical framework
The authors provide detailed articulation of conceptual frameworks and hypotheses developed iteratively as the review proceeds and in turn shaping the review and analysis. The review provides 'full-colour' illustrations of what the expert-authors judge to be key studies, key findings, key contradictions, and key gaps.

3. Transparency, quality appraisal and bias
This review includes little if any discussion about how the studies were identified and/or selected, but the approach would appear to have involved sampling for relevance rather than a systematic or exhaustive search. Similarly, there is no explicit discussion of study quality although an implicit hierarchy of evidence informs the review with longitudinal survey research presented as the 'gold standard'.

(continued overleaf)

Box 1.1   (continued)

---

4. A third order synthesis

The synthesis process adopted in this literature review resonates with many of the review approaches being developed today. For example, there are echoes of 'realist synthesis' (see Chapter 5) as the authors draw on various diverging sources of information with selection based on relevance and utility asking whether each source of evidence supports the hypothesis of interest or fits into the story they are developing. This process also resonates with the 'line of argument' approach elaborated by Noblit and Hare (1988) (see Chapter 4 on meta-ethnography). In the final chapter the authors explicitly note that they are going to draw on different stands to develop an over-arching argument about the story they are telling. The sources of evidence they draw on include:

- Statistical data
- Individual observational data collected in schools over three years
- Variables in their research and their indirect relationships to outcomes
- Findings from other research.

Rutter et al. go on to describe the process as a 'translation' of the research reviewed, echoing Noblit and Hare's meta-ethnography. Drawing on the evidence sources listed above, they develop the concept of 'school ethos' – and then consider how the individual process measures they have identified 'operate' in the context of a 'school ethos'. In this process they check out their results against findings of previous research. In general, in this process they seem to be looking for research (albeit not explicit or necessarily consciously) that confirms their ideas.

Second generation reviews

In recent years a 'second generation' of literature reviews has developed. These adopt to varying degrees the tenets of the systematic review (described below), notably following formal and transparent review processes; using explicit approaches to the identification and selection of evidence; and attending to the methodological quality of the studies included. Whilst they do not usually transform the evidence included into a common rubric, they explicitly seek to move beyond a thin description of the evidence to produce higher order syntheses resulting in the production of new knowledge and/or theory. An example of this type of literature review is the work by Greenhalgh et al. (2005) on organisational innovation, illustrated in Box 1.2. This review provides an account of how, why and in what sequence a field of research has unfolded, enabling the reader to see how explanations (theories) and empirical findings have intertwined and changed one another through time.

Box 1.2 A second generation literature review: the diffusion, spread and sustainability of innovations in service delivery organisations (Greenhalgh et al. 2005)

Exploratory searching and mapping of potentially relevant literature in a range of different areas by members of the research team from different disciplines (e.g. 'getting research into practice', 'diffusion of innovations in organisations', etc.) because of the size of the potentially relevant literature.

Feed back to other team members of examples of 'landmark' primary research papers in each of the different areas identified, which demonstrated the very wide range of different designs and theoretical orientations of studies undertaken over a forty-year period.

Revision of the original review question to: 'What research has been done that would help us understand the spread of innovations in organisations; what questions did the various research teams ask; and what did they find?'

Exploratory mapping showed that research on innovations tended to wax and wane within disciplines over time following 'break-through' pieces of research. The team decided to organise the review around '*research traditions*' which used different conceptual models of the diffusion of innovations and, within each, to identify how earlier work had led to later work using citation and reference tracking.

No single set of quality criteria, rather each study was judged according to the quality criteria relevant to the research tradition to which it belonged.

Initial presentation of findings on the spread of innovations in terms of 13 different 'research traditions' (e.g. those of rural sociology, evidence-based medicine and guideline implementation, communication studies and knowledge utilisation) each with its own landmark studies, core scientific paradigm (conceptual and methodological) and style of presentation which evolved over time (in contrast to an attempt at a comprehensive review).

Synthesis phase in which the findings from each research tradition were related to seven key dimensions of the spread and sustainability of innovations which crossed research traditions (e.g. innovations, adopters and adoption, communication and influence, organisational context, etc.).

Review able to identify many evidence-based options for spreading good ideas which could be tried in health services.

(continued overleaf)

Box 1.2 (continued)

Principles underlying this review

- Pragmatism – making judgments about inclusion during the review, rather than a priori
- Pluralism – response to the multi-disciplinary nature of the relevant literature
- Historicity – sequencing studies
- Contestation – between research traditions leads to attempt to find explanations that illuminate and challenge differences in findings and recommendations from different traditions.
- Peer review – emerging findings constantly tested by others inside and outside the research team

---

The strengths and limitations of literature reviews

Dixon-Woods and colleagues (2004) have argued that literature, or 'narrative' reviews as they called them, are flexible, allowing for the inclusion of different types of evidence – qualitative and quantitative, research and non-research. This flexibility and ease of handling of a wide range of evidence means that such approaches are likely to remain an important tool for policy- and management-relevant reviews. Although the majority of these types of review still do not follow standardised procedures, as the example in Figure 2.2 illustrates, an increasing number are tending towards greater formality and explicitness in the drive for increased transparency and rigour in evidence review. At the very least, this entails paying attention to the methodological quality of the studies reviewed, and to wider issues of validity, such as the adequacy of findings (see Chapter 2 for a more detailed consideration of quality appraisal).

Both the limitations and the conceptual and analytical sophistication that can be achieved by first generation literature reviews were illustrated by the review of anti-social behaviour research undertaken by Rutter and colleagues (1998; see Box 1.1). However, as Pawson and Bellaby (2006) have argued it would be wrong to assume that the lack of standardised methods inevitably means that there is no logic to the methods used in traditional literature reviews. They suggest that literature reviews, for example those focusing on whether particular programmes or interventions work, are based on a relatively complex 'configurational approach to causality'.

> According to this perspective narrative reviews of evidence on the effectiveness of programmes or interventions are built on the assumption that positive outcomes will result from the combination of a series of program/intervention attributes ... Interventions work, it is considered, because of the compatibility of target group, setting,

program stratagem, program content, implementation details, stake-holder alliances and so on. When using this framework it is the entire 'recipe' that makes the difference. All of these ingredients, along with information on outcomes and on the methodology employed in the original evaluations constitute the ontology (or the how), of narrative review.

(Pawson and Bellaby 2006: 85)

From this perspective, the task of the reviewer is to identify studies that provide the richest description of the significant properties of a particular programme or intervention. Literature reviews can be used to identify examples of 'good practice' or 'best buys' based on a judgment of the 'fit' between an intervention or programme and the critical success factors the review has identified.

There are practical challenges associated with traditional literature review. Their very flexibility means that the number of studies and other sources that can potentially be included could become unmanageable as could the amount of information to be extracted from studies. Additionally, diversity in the type of research makes the appraisal of study quality difficult, presents particular problems for the extraction of data in a common format and makes it hard to weight different types of evidence.

Perhaps the most important criticism of literature reviews is the potential for bias and hence for unreliable conclusions to be drawn. Shadish and colleagues (1991) suggest that in order to claim generalisability literature reviews have to demonstrate 'proximal similarity'. This process involves selecting a feasible number of studies to review rather than attempting to be comprehensive, and choosing a manageable number of programme characteristics to explore in detail from what would certainly be a much larger number. Pawson and Bellaby question the logic of 'proximal similarity', suggesting that in this process some studies and factors will be privileged over others and that this introduces a whole range of biases – from those associated with publications to those arising from the personal orientation and interests of the reviewer. However, the extent to which this problem is unique to literature reviews should not be exaggerated. Recent debates in quantitative meta-analysis of trials of effectiveness have often turned on which studies to include and how much weight to give to each (Mayor 2001; Olsen and Gøtzche 2001).

Systematic reviews of effectiveness

Systematic reviews of health care effectiveness developed out of a need to review health research evidence and the desire for an explicit, transparent, reproducible method for this. The systematic review is a method used to summarise, appraise and synthesize high quality evidence on effectiveness. A review is generally described as systematic if it has these features:

- a review protocol to guide the review process
- comprehensive literature searching using a pre-defined search strategy
- critical appraisal of studies and grading of evidence
- explicit (transparent) inclusion and exclusion criteria
- explicit (transparent) data extraction
- explicit (typically statistical) analysis.

In addition, it is increasingly expected that systematic reviews will be regularly updated. As has already been noted, some of these features designed to ensure that the review is systematic and avoids bias are also found in 'second generation' literature reviews. However, an important characteristic of systematic reviews (see Cochrane reviews, below) is that the process followed is largely linear and preordained, for example, the review question or the data included cannot be altered on the basis of emerging findings or analysis of the evidence. Some approaches to synthesis, and to reviewing more generally, have a less linear, more iterative process and this can be the source of some tension between the different approaches to reviewing.

In the world of health research, systematic reviews are closely allied to the evidence-based medicine movement which has, more recently, extended to encompass policy and professional practice more broadly. In 1972, a lecture by the epidemiologist Archie Cochrane (Cochrane 1972) was published which berated medical practice as ineffective and at worst harmful to patients. He advocated the use of randomised controlled trial (RCT) methods to test the effects of interventions and argued that the findings from such trials should form the basis of decisions about practice, and perhaps more importantly decisions about health care priorities and funding: only those treatments shown to be effective should be funded. The RCT has become widely accepted as the best method for evaluating effectiveness within Cochrane systematic reviews. Cochrane also attacked the medical profession for failing adequately to summarise or collect the findings of existing RCTs. This spawned various efforts by individuals and organisations to collect and review RCTs of health care interventions. One of the earliest attempts to address the lack of knowledge about effectiveness was led by Chalmers and colleagues (1989) who spent a decade or more first producing a database of effective interventions in pregnancy and childbirth, and then testing methods for synthesizing the results from multiple studies. Efforts to develop systematic reviews have led to the creation of worldwide organisations such as the Cochrane and Campbell Collaborations which collect and review research evidence on the effectiveness of health and other social policy interventions (see Box 1.3) and to the development of resources such as the Cochrane Library of Systematic Reviews.

Interest in reviewing evidence grew during the late 1970s particularly in the USA in the field of education and by the 1980s the technique of

---

Box 1.3 The Cochrane and Campbell collaborations, and the UK NHS Centre for Reviews and Dissemination

---

The UK Cochrane Centre was established at the end of 1992, by the National Health Service Research and Development Programme. 'to facilitate and co-ordinate the preparation and maintenance of systematic reviews of randomized controlled trials of health care'. The UK Cochrane Centre is now one of twelve Cochrane Centres around the world which provide the infrastructure for co-ordinating The Cochrane Collaboration. The Cochrane Collaboration was founded in 1993 and named after the British epidemiologist, Archie Cochrane. The Cochrane Collaboration is an international non-profit and independent organisation, dedicated to making up-to-date, accurate information about the effects of health care readily available worldwide. It produces and disseminates systematic reviews of health care interventions and promotes the search for evidence in the form of clinical trials and other studies of interventions.
http://www.cochrane.co.uk/en/collaboration.htm accessed 27/10/06

The more recent international Campbell Collaboration (established in 1999) pre-pares, maintains and disseminates systematic reviews of studies of interventions in areas of social policy other than health care, such as education, welfare and policing and prisons. It acquires and promotes access to information about trials of interventions and builds summaries and electronic brochures of reviews and reports of trials for policy makers, practitioners, researchers and the public.
http://www.campbellcollaboration.org/ accessed 27/10/06

The UK Centre for Reviews and Dissemination (CRD) was established in January 1994, with funding from the English Department of Health and aims to pro-vide research-based information about the effects of interventions used in health and social care. It helps to promote the use of research-based knowledge, by undertaking systematic reviews on selected topics and scoping reviews of the research literature; maintaining databases of reviews; and disseminating guidance about best practice methods for systemic reviews including, of late, reviewing qualitative research.
http://www.york.ac.uk/inst/crd/aboutcrd.htm accessed 27/10/06

---

meta-analysis was established for aggregating statistical findings (Glass et al. 1981; Hunter and Schmidt 2004). Meta-analysis is a statistical technique used to summarise effect size from similar quantitative studies by pooling their results. Pooling the results of quantitative studies increases the statistical power of the analysis (e.g. of the relative effectiveness of two different treatments for the same condition) to detect even small effects: the more studies that can be pooled, the greater the precision of the estimate of effect. Meta-analysis also enabled analysts to investigate the reasons for statistical variations between studies to see to what extent these were due to chance. Powered by such methods, systematic reviewing proliferated in the 1980s and 1990s and was increasingly seen as a resource not just for evidence-based medicine, but for the wider realms of public policy- and decision-making (Davies et al. 2000).

Systematic reviews of effectiveness are based on the assumption that there is a hierarchy of evidence (Box 1.4) – that some forms of evidence are 'better', or more valuable than others. From this viewpoint, systematic reviews of effectiveness are seen as carrying greater weight than a single study. This has been the subject of a great deal of debate and controversy with some commentators arguing that it is inappropriate to extend the notion of evidence hierarchies beyond questions of effectiveness.

Moving beyond effectiveness reviews

It is increasingly recognised that the hierarchy of evidence applies principally to effectiveness reviews and is less appropriate for wider reviewing activities. Whilst the more complex questions asked by policy- and decision-makers often include a concern with effectiveness (where the hierarchy may be relevant) they move well beyond this focus. Moreover there is a growing consensus (see for example Popay and Williams 1998; Petticrew and Roberts 2005) that methods for evidence review and synthesis have to be tailored to review questions. For the more complex questions facing policy- and decision-makers (see Box 1.5) a myriad of other forms of evidence in the widest sense – including qualitative research, non-trial based quantitative research, views of stakeholders and expert panels – will potentially be relevant. So, for example, research in Canada shows that health authority decision-makers take a broad and pragmatic view of what constitutes relevant evidence for

---

Box 1.4   The evidence hierarchy for effectiveness reviews

- Systematic reviews and meta-analysis
- RCTs
- Quasi experimental designs – cohort studies, case-control studies
- Surveys
- Case reports
- Qualitative methods
- Anecdote/expert or user opinion

Box 1.5   Questions that can confront policy-makers, managers and patients

- In what sense is this a 'problem';
- How and why has it come about;
- How significant is it compared to other problems on the policy or management agenda;
- How is it changing over time;
- What is likely to work to address the problem,
- . . . for whom and under what circumstances;
- What if any are the differential impacts of interventions across social groups;
- How cost-effective are different policy/management options likely to be in the current context;
- How do the different options work; and
- how acceptable are different interventions to target groups, the wider population and providers?

---

priority-setting, including non-randomised quantitative studies, qualitative research, expert opinion and other more subjective sources such as anecdotal reports (Mitton and Patten 2004).

Many systematic reviews, including those following the Cochrane model attempt to answer the wider questions that policy-makers typically ask. As a result, there is greater recognition of the contribution of diverse kinds of evidence, notably qualitative research evidence. This is partly linked to the growing acceptability and recognised utility of these methods in primary health-related research where qualitative methods are increasingly used alongside quantitative methods on the grounds that the two sets of data can be complementary or interactive, with the findings of one prompting questions and lines of analysis for the other (O'Cathain and Thomas 2006). The same logic potentially applies to reviews but is less apparent perhaps because methods for incorporating qualitative research and other evidence in systematic reviews are relatively underdeveloped and present a major methodological and practical developmental challenge (Dixon-Woods et al. 2001; Harden et al. 2004).

Different objectives of reviews – 'knowledge support' versus 'decision support'

A lot of the debate about the appropriate scope of evidence that is legitimate to include in systematic reviews arises because of confusion about the purpose of different reviews. As well as recognising that the evidence and methods used for a review should relate to the questions to be answered, it is worth understanding the different objectives of reviews. It is particularly helpful to distinguish between reviews that aim to provide 'knowledge support' and those that attempt to provide 'decision support' (Dowie 2001; Mays et al. 2005). It is important to establish which of these objectives a review seeks to meet at the outset. A review for knowledge support will be confined to summarising and synthesizing research evidence whereas the decision support function is served by a review that also includes some or all of the remaining analytical tasks required to reach a decision in a particular context.

A knowledge support review could be undertaken to answer the question 'What does the qualitative and quantitative research evidence tell us about adherence to medication by patients with asthma?' This might entail the following supplementary questions (Greenhalgh et al. 2004a):

- What do we know about the rates of adherence to different medications for this disease?
- Why do patients take or not take their medicines?
- Is there anything 'special' or unusual about asthma that might make adherence different in some way for these patients?
- Are there any population characteristics to consider (e.g. age, socioeconomic class or racial differences) that could affect adherence?
- What techniques have been tried to increase adherence to asthma medicines?
- Is adherence an acceptable or shared goal for patients and their health care providers?

These types of question can be quite broad. By contrast the kinds of question suited to decision support type reviews are likely to be much more focused and specific. A decision support review question might be 'Should the UK NHS invest more in cognitive behavioural therapy (CBT) for people with bipolar disorders?' Such a review would need to go beyond effectiveness questions to ask, for example:

- Does CBT work?
- Do other treatments also work?
- Which treatment works best?
- Is CBT cost-effective compared with other treatments?
- What level of improvement is shown in patients undergoing CBT and is it sufficient to alter people's lives (e.g. so that they can return to work or normal activities)?
- How much is currently spent on CBT and how is it spent in the UK?
- How much of the existing spending could be better spent?
- What are the resource implications of investing in CBT for all the

patients who currently do not receive it but who could benefit cost-effectively?

- How acceptable would CBT be to the people at whom it would be targeted?
- What are the competing priorities in mental health care and more widely?
- What are the supply issues related to such investment (i.e. staff and facilities)?
- How feasible is it to increase CBT capacity?

The distinction between knowledge and decision support has major implications for the choice of approach to reviewing and within this to the method for synthesizing evidence. Systematic reviews designed to support policy decision-making may use more than one synthesis method within the same review. For example, a systematic review may include quantitative evidence of the effectiveness of different interventions using statistical meta-analysis, alongside a qualitative (and non-statistical) synthesis of the qualitative research evidence of their acceptability. The function of the review will influence the research questions and is likely to lead to a differing emphasis on qualitative and quantitative evidence; the more a review aims to contribute directly to a specific decision, the more it is likely to have to include non-research evidence as well as methods of modelling and simulation (see below).

Synthesis

Evidence synthesis embodies the idea, contained in the dictionary definition (Box 1.6) of making a new whole out of the parts: individual studies or pieces of evidence are somehow combined to produce a coherent whole, in the form of an argument, theory or conclusions. Synthesis is thus a distinct element in the review process. When the process of undertaking a systematic review is represented in linear form, synthesis is viewed as an activity at or close to the end of the review process. It occurs once the evidence has been accumulated and the data of interest extracted (see Box 1.7 overleaf).

Box 1.6   A definition of synthesis

Synthesis *noun*. Building up; putting together; making a whole out of parts; the combination of separate elements of thought into a whole; reasoning from principles to a conclusion (opp. to *analysis*). Chambers Dictionary, 1992.

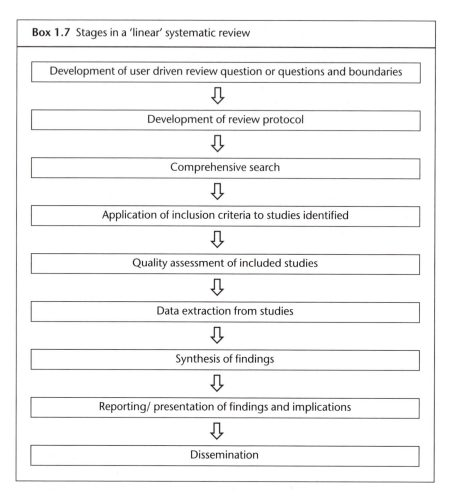

Box 1.7 Stages in a 'linear' systematic review

Development of user driven review question or questions and boundaries

⇩

Development of review protocol

⇩

Comprehensive search

⇩

Application of inclusion criteria to studies identified

⇩

Quality assessment of included studies

⇩

Data extraction from studies

⇩

Synthesis of findings

⇩

Reporting/ presentation of findings and implications

⇩

Dissemination

Hammersley distinguishes three meanings for the word synthesis in the context of systematic reviews. First it can mean 'aggregative' – that is focused on the cumulation and generalisation of evidence (as in the Cochrane and Campbell collaborations); second it can mean comparative or 'replicative' – that is focused on the extent to which different sources of evidence reinforce one another by comparison between sources); and third it can mean that the review focused on developing 'theory' or explanations (Hammersley 2006: 240–1). Systematic reviews are often seen as aggregative by researchers and policy-makers/managers, but the developmental role of reviews may be equally important, for example, in generating early policy ideas or theories that can inform the development of new interventions with a plausible change mechanism underpinning them. The developmental role of reviews is particularly associated with approaches to synthesis such as realist reviews (see Chapter 5) and meta-ethnography (see Chapter 4) but all forms of synthesis could make this type of contribution if reviewers designed these aims into the review.

There are a number of different approaches to synthesis that have potential to be applied to varied research evidence and may also have potential to be used for the review of non-research sources of evidence. However, practical experience and good examples of specific methods are limited, in some cases to a single exemplar. Most of the methods for synthesis discussed in this book were developed for primary research data analysis rather than for synthesizing research evidence. Of the methods available, most were developed either for synthesizing qualitative or quantitative research evidence rather than for combining the two in a single synthesis. However it is hoped that presenting and discussing the potential application of these methods in this book will encourage further attempts to synthesize qualitative and quantitative evidence, and persuade reviewers to explore ways of combining and integrating different kinds of evidence to inform policy- and decision-making and to contribute to the further development of methods in this field.

Noblit and Hare (1988) make a useful distinction between 'interpretive' and 'integrative' forms of synthesis which relates to the nature of the synthesis rather than the use to which it will be put (i.e. knowledge or decision support). Interpretive synthesis combines evidence by seeking to develop new concepts and theories (interpretations). Integrative synthesis can be seen as focusing on collecting and summarising data, (i.e. 'knowledge accumulation') although these approaches may also produce new knowledge through a 'meta-analysis' for example that provides a new estimate of the direction and size of effect. Borrowing from Hammersley's typology of synthesis Dixon-Woods et al. (2006a: 36) have proposed substituting the term aggregative synthesis for integrative synthesis. 'Aggregative synthesis' is a term that could be applied to many literature reviews and systematic reviews, whereas the emphasis on interpretation in interpretive synthesis has meant that these approaches have largely been associated with the synthesis of qualitative research findings (see Chapter 4).

Is it feasible to synthesize disparate evidence?

There is considerable controversy about the legitimacy and/or feasibility of combining the findings of different types of evidence, notably evidence from different kinds of research. Within the qualitative research community, in particular, it is suggested that attempts at aggregative synthesis destroy the integrity of individual studies thereby producing meaningless findings (Sandelowski et al. 1997). This critique is informed by a relatively extreme 'relativist' position which argues that qualitative research offers multiple 'truths' or realities such that each study represents a unique, personalised view that cannot be replicated, added to another or transferred. This argument is further complicated when a synthesis attempts to combine findings across different methods or studies informed by different theories of knowledge: relativists, for example, would suggest that differences in theory and method are fundamental and militate against any integration of research. However, a 'subtle realist' view (Hammersley 1992) would suggest that while there may well be multiple descriptions or explanations of phenomena and ways of knowing, these ultimately relate to some underlying reality or truth. From this perspective, synthesis is accepted as potentially promoting a greater understanding than any single study could achieve.

There are those who contend that the divide between the qualitative and quantitative research paradigms is far greater than the differences between different types of qualitative research, and that this is an irremovable barrier to the synthesis of qualitative and quantitative evidence. However, to some extent this divide between qualitative and quantitative research is being bridged in primary studies as many researchers now engage productively in multi-method research, utilising both quantitative and qualitative methods (O'Cathain and Thomas 2006). Synthesis may be seen as a logical extension of this combined approach. Just as in mixed method primary research, qualitative data can illuminate why a particular policy or management approach has variable impacts and suggest ways of dealing with this, and quantitative studies can indicate its relative effectiveness overall: both have a contribution to make to understanding the processes shaping implementation of interventions/programmes.

The feasibility of synthesizing non-research evidence has been little explored but similar issues arise regarding the context and applicability of non-research evidence and these are overlaid with concerns about validity and rigour. Nonetheless, these forms of evidence may well be necessary components of decision-making in messy, complex policy arenas and the question here may be less 'is it feasible to synthesize these kinds of evidence?' and more 'is it legitimate to ignore them?'

Evidence synthesis can help to inform decision-making by managers and policy-makers. It can answer questions which individual studies or other pieces of evidence cannot – by integrating and interpreting complex and diverse kinds of evidence in a form which is more manageable and accessible. Used for knowledge support synthesis can inform – identifying gaps where further research is needed, locating controversy and mapping the terrain. In a decision support mode, synthesis can be used to help decide between competing priorities or alternatives.

The next chapter looks in more detail at the process of reviewing evidence systematically to provide the foundation for synthesis.

2 Stages in reviewing evidence systematically

This chapter looks at the main elements in reviewing evidence and how the process of conducting a review can be approached, structured and reported in a way that makes these elements rigorous and transparent. Although the format of this chapter presents the various elements as if they occur in succession, it is likely that a review examining questions that extend beyond the effectiveness of policies or interventions will be undertaken more iteratively. In these cases, the review process is seldom linear, some elements taking place in parallel, and others being revisited and further developed as the review progresses. As later chapters of the book show, many approaches to evidence synthesis are also iterative and this calls for some flexibility regarding how different phases of a review are undertaken and how the review process as a whole is approached.

A guiding principle in all approaches to systematic reviewing and synthesis is to be as rigorous and as transparent as possible. One way of being transparent is to draft a protocol near the start of a review, as for a primary study, setting out the questions and methods of the review, including how studies will be searched for, assessed and synthesized. This protocol will be adapted as the review process unfolds, but it is helpful to have some structure from the outset. This chapter provides a template for structuring the review process that can be used to guide the development of a review protocol and inform the conduct of a synthesis. Before looking in detail at the elements involved in undertaking a review this chapter briefly revisits the question 'what is the review for?' since the answer has a major effect on how the review is carried out.

Reviews for decision support and reviews for knowledge support

Systematic reviews of effectiveness are often conducted because of uncertainty about the impact of interventions, for example, to see if the evidence indicates that a particular drug or treatment works in the management of a particular disease. However, as already noted, the concerns of policy-makers, managers, practitioners and service users often go beyond effectiveness and as a result the questions asked by these decision-makers tend to be very broadly expressed, for example they might include:

- How important is childhood obesity as a public health issue? Should we do anything about it?
- What is the best way to manage depression – drugs, cognitive behavioural therapy or something else?
- Which element in the government's early childhood programme appears to contribute the most to the outcomes observed and should it be expanded?
- Is it the right policy goal to increase the number of 18-year-olds entering higher education?
- Why do certain people not use public transport and how can we encourage them to do so?
- Should I have the treatment recommended to me or are there alternative ways of managing my condition?

This list shows that decision-makers often need to know more than the answer to the question 'does x work?' and 'does it work better than y?' They may on occasions need to know how x works and why its effect seems to vary in some settings and with certain social groups rather than others. They may need to know why it works better in association with other programmes or interventions. They may also need to know whether x is likely to be acceptable to the public. At the outset, they may need to know whether a specific problem matters (how important is it and what are its consequences likely to be?). Sometimes a review is undertaken simply to provide an overview of a body of literature. For example, before paying for new research, a research funding body might commission reviews or expect research applicants to provide them, focusing on questions such as:

- What does qualitative research evidence tell us about how people use medicines?
- What is known about 'help-seeking behaviour' in relation to people's health?

All of these kinds of question require access to complex and multi-faceted sources of evidence. The answers are likely to be found in diverse places, sometimes traversing studies that generate both qualitative and quantitative findings, sometimes drawing on other forms of 'intelligence' such as expert opinion or stakeholder views. In answering these kinds of question it will therefore be necessary to synthesize material from different studies and sources.

In Chapter 1 it was suggested, in very broad terms, that reviews could be seen as providing either 'decision support' or 'knowledge support'. It is important to establish at the outset which of these purposes will underpin the review. Synthesis can form part of a review for either knowledge or decision support, but knowledge support tends to be confined to summarising the scientific research evidence, while decision support includes some or all of the remaining analytical tasks required to reach a decision in a policy or management context. It is vital that the objective is clarified and agreed because it affects the choice of approaches to synthesis and decisions about what type of evidence to include in the review: ideally this is something that the review team and the commissioners or users of a review should discuss and agree in advance.

Where a review aims to contribute directly to a specific decision, it is likely that policy-makers will need to be either members of the review team or, at least, closely involved in the process (e.g. ensuring that the team has access to the necessary 'soft' evidence relevant to the particular decision). The decision support versus knowledge support distinction also has implications for the skill-mix required by the review team. Again, in the case of reviews for decision support it may be necessary to derive a professional, 'expert', political or public consensus on an issue where research findings are lacking by applying formal methods of consensus development e.g. Delphi, nominal group or citizens' jury techniques (Black et al. 1998; Black 2006).

The purpose of the review will also determine the research questions and this, in turn, may lead to a differing emphasis on qualitative and quantitative evidence. Where a review aims to provide decision support it may need to include non-research evidence and possibly use various methods of modelling and simulation (e.g. to link what is known from research to data or assumptions relevant to the specific setting of the decision which the research cannot supply). The purpose will also affect the methodological focus. In reviews for knowledge support, approaches which avoid bias may be prioritised, whereas for decision support avoidance of bias may be necessary, but not sufficient since the reviewer must also be explicit about the basis of the judgements inevitably made. The purpose may further affect the audience or users of the review. Often the audience for knowledge support reviews will be other researchers, but decision support reviews need to be accessible to a less specialist audience of those directly involved in specific decisions, such as policy-makers and managers.

Stages or elements in a systematic review

The process of undertaking a systematic review of the effectiveness of a policy or intervention for 'knowledge support' has been well documented (Chalmers et al. 1993; Chalmers and Altman 1995; Petticrew and Roberts 2006) and the broad features of such reviews were outlined in Chapter 1. The main elements in a systematic review of effectiveness are usually presented as occurring in strict sequence (as in Box 1.7, p. 17). However, outside the Cochrane Collaboration model of systematic reviewing, the reality of the review process is often acknowledged to be less linear than this model implies. Rather, the process contains opportunities to backtrack, to revisit, for example, the protocol, or to develop theory at different moments – as the model in Figure 2.1 illustrates. Keeping this iterative model in mind, but in an attempt to provide some structure for a review (and a way to locate synthesis), the following sections of this chapter describe the principal elements in the review process in a linear manner.

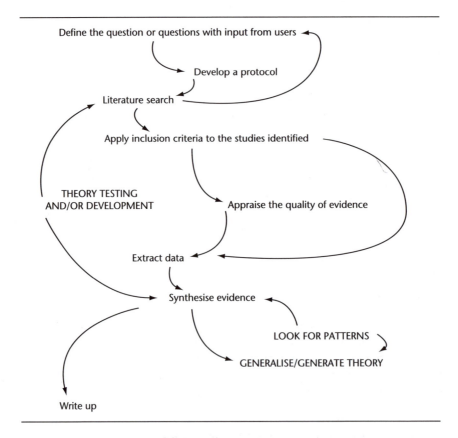

Figure 2.1 An iterative view of the review process.

Defining the question or questions

This element includes the development of the review question(s) (ideally in consultation with likely end users and/or commissioners) preliminary mapping or scoping of the evidence which informs this developmental work and eventual specification of the question or questions.

The review question has to be both relevant to potential users of the review and, in theory at least, answerable – sometimes this can be a tricky balance to achieve. In the context of policy and management decision-making, review questions should be developed iteratively at or near the beginning of the review process. This is likely to be based on discussion between the relevant decision-makers/commissioners and the reviewers as they begin to examine the evidence, and as they learn more about the policy environment in which the review is to be used. These discussions will also need to consider why the issue is on the policy/management agenda and how the review is likely to be used. However, just as in much primary research, additional or amended questions are likely to emerge from the process of collecting and analysing the data. In one recent, systematic review of both qualitative and quantitative evidence, all the questions were developed from the process of reading and re-reading the articles retrieved, rather than a priori (Garcia et al. 2002).

Often the initial questions are broad and multi-faceted, for example, a pressing question from a manager or policy-maker might be: 'What are the costs, benefits and quality impacts of integrated health care delivery systems (with or without physician integration) compared with non-integrated delivery systems?' To be feasible as a question for a review, time would need to be spent agreeing a definition of 'integration' and perhaps also deciding to focus on particular services to make the scope of the review more manageable. A policy-maker's question such as: 'Should the government allow private magnetic resonance imaging (MRI) facilities?' has either to be recast to focus on the costs and benefits of public versus private MRI, if it is to be answered for the purpose of 'knowledge support', or if the review is to contribute to a decision as to whether or not to permit private MRI in a particular setting, the reviewers would need access to non-research evidence such as some indication of the trade-offs ministers were willing to make between, say, equity, quality, cost and efficiency in the particular country or regional context.

In some instances the review question can be clearly delineated at an early stage. More often, however, whilst an initial focus for the review can be identified, a 'mapping' of the available relevant evidence needs to be carried out before the specific question or questions for the review can be specified (c.f. Oliver et al. 2005). This is particularly likely to be the case in areas that have not been reviewed systematically before and/or where the evidence is widely scattered across different disciplines and fields of endeavour.

A mapping exercise can be used to assess the need for a systematic review and/or to guide and refine the scope of the review. It is especially useful in situations where a broad question is of interest, such as: 'How effective are interventions to prevent unintentional injuries?'; or 'What do we know about the factors that enable or constrain changes in clinical practice?' By mapping the available literature addressing the latter broad question it is possible to:

- describe the types of interventions that have been evaluated or the focus of studies that have looked at factors shaping clinical behaviour change, together with the sorts of study designs used
- see if anyone else has done a review, narrative or otherwise, in this field
- assess the volume and distribution of potentially relevant literature.

Based on this initial mapping, reviewers working with potential users of the review (including commissioners/funders) can refine the scope of the review so that the questions to be addressed are both answerable and relevant. Some reviewers establish advisory groups to support them in this process and throughout the rest of the review. The results of the mapping process should also help with determining how much time the review is likely to take and the sorts of disciplinary skill needed in the review team.

The search for studies during a mapping stage will usually be wide-ranging. It is likely to involve a variety of electronic databases relevant to the topic of the review. Other sources may also be searched, including conference proceedings, websites, personal contact with researchers in the field, hand-searching of specialist journals and databases (for example databases of 'grey' or unpublished literature), and scanning of reference lists from studies already identified. This wider and more time-consuming searching can be left until potentially relevant studies identified through electronic databases have been described and decisions made about the exact question(s) for review. An obvious starting point for the mapping stage is to search for existing reviews, systematic or not, by looking, for instance, in databases of reviews such as that of the Campbell Collaboration in social policy or the Cochrane Collaboration Database of Systematic Reviews in the health field (see http://www.camp bellcollaboration.org/ and http://www.cochrane.co.uk/en/collaboration.htm).

Getting the question right takes time. In the context of systematic reviews of effectiveness the PICO acronym helps to focus attention on the four key components of a well-formulated question: the People (or participants) who are the focus of the interventions; the Interventions; the Comparison(s); and the Outcomes (Booth and Fry-Smith 2004, see Figure 2.2). Sometimes a fifth component that relates to type of study design or context/setting is also included. For reviews within the social sciences the SPICE acronym – Setting,

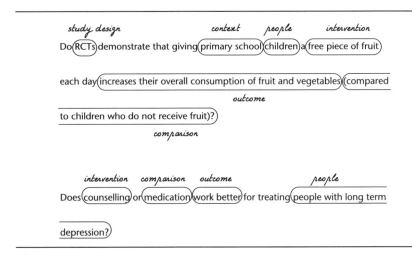

study design   *context*   *people*   *intervention*
Do RCTs demonstrate that giving primary school children a free piece of fruit

each day increases their overall consumption of fruit and vegetables (compared
                                                  outcome

to children who do not receive fruit)?
          comparison

    intervention   *comparison*   *outcome*   *people*
Does counselling or medication work better for treating people with long term

depression?

Figure 2.2 Examples of effectiveness questions.

Perspective, Intervention (or problem of Interest) Comparison and Evaluation has been proposed by Booth (2004) and serves a similar function.

In theory the types of questions that can be addressed by evidence reviews are endless but in the context of policy decision-making Harden and Thomas (2005) suggest there are three very different types of question that systematic reviews can address. They include questions that may contribute to the development of new interventions to address a particular policy- or practice-relevant issue; questions about the feasibility of implementing interventions already shown to be effective in an experimental situation; and the more 'traditional' effectiveness questions including, for example, questions concerning the balance between benefits and harm associated with particular interventions and the factors that determine this balance. Examples of questions that underpin these reviews are shown in Box 2.1.

Box 2.1   Examples of review questions from recent reviews

- What does the literature on innovations have to tell us about the spread and sustainability of innovations in health service delivery and organisations? (Greenhalgh et al. 2004a)
- What is known about the barriers, to and facilitators of, health and health behaviours among young people? (Shepherd et al. 2006)
- What do the qualitative and quantitative research literatures tell us about access to health care by vulnerable, socio-economically disadvantaged people in the UK? (Dixon-Woods et al. 2005)

The review question helps to locate and select studies for inclusion in the review. While the reviewer often needs to retain flexibility to develop the question as part of the iterative process of conducting the review, poorly specified questions can lead to difficulties in deciding which studies should be included and which excluded. There has been considerable debate about whether review questions should be broad or narrow in scope – there are advantages to both approaches, but the key point is that the review question has to be answerable, and relevant to the review users.

Determining the types of study to be included

Once the review question has been agreed, the key components of the question (i.e. people, intervention, comparison, outcomes and context) can be used to select studies for inclusion on the basis of relevance and/or study type. It is usually necessary to elaborate on the key components to aid this selection process and make sure that decisions made are transparent to users of the review. This also means that somebody else could reproduce the review if necessary, for instance to update the review and to add new studies – although in the context of an interpretative synthesis process this does not necessarily mean that the precise findings of the review will be reproducible.

Thus, for example, in a review of the effectiveness of interventions for preventing unintentional injuries in children, the reviewer would obviously incorporate studies which include children. But s/he must also decide if the review will include studies focusing on children of all ages, or just children between certain ages, or whether the review will focus only on specific groups of children, such as those at high risk of injury. There will also be decisions to be made about the type of interventions; for example, will the review include studies of any intervention aimed at preventing unintentional injuries, or only certain types of interventions (for example, multi-faceted community based interventions, as opposed to those focusing more narrowly on interventions in schools)? If the reviewer intends to synthesize evidence on the implementation of an intervention, s/he might want to specify which of the many different types of factor/process that could influence implementation s/he will include. The review could, for example, focus on specific aspects of organisational structure and culture, and/or professional competencies and skills, as well as factors associated with the people and/or communities at whom the intervention is targeted. Reviewers may also wish to include evidence from the perspective of people who are the 'target' of particular interventions – to explore their experience of the intervention under consideration, or more generally their perspectives on their needs and how they feel they are best met. Similarly, the reviewer would need to define the outcomes of interest. For example, the outcomes of injury prevention will have been measured in a variety of ways across different studies.

As noted in Chapter 1 the idea of a hierarchy of evidence is problematic in reviews that move beyond narrowly defined questions of effectiveness. Decisions about which types of study and kinds of evidence to include depend on the purpose of the review and the question(s) it seeks to answer. Rather than thinking in terms of a hierarchy of study designs, it is better to think of a process of matching types of evidence to particular questions on the basis of their relevance and validity when used to answer specific questions. More anecdotal or impressionistic material may be helpful as background (e.g. when formulating the questions for the review), but is less likely to be included systematically in bibliographic databases. If the aim of a review is primarily to develop theory for subsequent testing, then there may be few objections (other than practicality) to the use of a wide range of 'evidence' as in 'realist synthesis' (see Chapter 5). Similarly, if the purpose of the review is to contribute directly to a specific decision in a particular context (rather than providing knowledge support), then it is almost certainly going to be necessary to assemble other kinds of evidence alongside formal research-based evidence (e.g. country-specific expert opinion or the values policy-makers place on achieving particular outcomes).

In areas where there is likely to be a large amount of literature, it will be important to consider the breadth of evidence to be included. In the context of effectiveness reviews, this issue has been referred to as 'lumping and splitting' (Petticrew and Roberts 2006: 48–9) The rationale for adopting a broad approach (lumping) is to be able to identify common, generalised features of the effect of interventions across different settings. As a result small differences in study characteristics may not be of crucial importance. This is contrasted with the rationale for adopting a narrower approach (splitting) which is used to explore differences. 'Splitters' specify that it is appropriate to include only studies that are similar in terms of design, population, interventions and outcomes (Grimshaw et al. 2003). Both approaches are valid. Policy-makers tend to approach researchers with 'lumping' questions and researchers mostly prefer to answer narrower questions resulting from 'splitting'.

There is some debate about whether to sample when there is a large body of literature and there are too many sources of evidence to be reviewed feasibly. No 'best' method has been proposed for such sampling should it be needed. Undertaking a 'review of reviews' when there is more than one review available may be one option if time or resources are constrained, ideally accompanied by a search for studies published since the latest review. The English Health Development Agency, now subsumed into the National Institute for Health and Clinical Excellence (NICE) commissioned a number of such reviews, which are well regarded in the health promotion field (e.g. Kelly et al. 2004). These may be particularly suitable when there is lack of time to commission an external team and the review is undertaken in-house. However, if the existing reviews are predominately unsystematic literature reviews they may well not be particularly representative of the field of interest.

Sampling is beginning to be discussed in relation to reviews of research, though in the context of systematic reviews of effectiveness, the emphasis in the influential Cochrane Collaboration has been on including, as far as possible, all the RCTs in an area, including unpublished studies in order to overcome publication bias. There is clearly a tension between minimising the potential for publication bias and making reviews (particularly 'lumpy' ones) manageable. Reviews that involve the transformation of raw data, or that include large numbers of studies, require greater resources, and where the review question and/or range of evidence is very broad, it may be necessary to sample. In relation to qualitative studies, and arguably some quantitative or mixed method research and non-research sources of evidence, the main choice is between some form of purposive sampling (i.e. in which studies are sampled according to a set of characteristics such as size, setting and design) or theoretical sampling in which studies are selected for their relevance in testing a particular theory or explanation for a phenomenon. In both cases, the concept of 'saturation' familiar to qualitative researchers in primary studies, in which data are collected until no new issues are identified, could be applied to reviews so that studies would be included until the latest studies ceased to provide any fresh data or insights. Another approach where a review is deliberately broad (e.g. because the area has not been reviewed before) is to confine the systematic part of the review to one of the questions (e.g. on effectiveness) and to use a less comprehensive approach to other questions because of the difficulty of determining inclusions/exclusions (e.g. when outlining policy debates surrounding the implementation of an intervention).

There is the further issue of how much information from a study or other source (i.e. reference, abstract or full text of papers) is necessary before any decision can be made about inclusion or exclusion. Frequently, the final set of decisions can be made only with reference to the full text of papers. There are also debates, particularly in relation to reviews of qualitative research about whether an inclusion or exclusion decision is appropriate at all, particularly in the early phase of a review. One study (Pound et al. 2005) used two simple 'screening' questions about the relevance of the study to the topic and whether it used qualitative data and analysis to determine initial inclusion. During the synthesis stage of this study further identified papers were excluded for a variety of reasons, for example because their conceptual framework was fundamentally incompatible with the other studies in the synthesis.

An alternative approach is to collect the literature and undertake quality appraisal of studies in order to be able to give different weights to different sources of evidence during the synthesis process but without necessarily excluding studies. This approach is supported by the SUMARI software developed by the Joanna Briggs Institute (www.joannabriggs.edu.au) (see Chapter 6) which contains a quality appraisal tool and a mechanism for ranking each piece of evidence in terms of three levels of credibility. However, this approach has significant resource and time implications if there is a large relevant literature and there is also a debate about the feasibility of such a technical approach to methodological quality appraisal in qualitative research. More details about inclusion and exclusion criteria are provided later in this chapter.

Comprehensive literature searching

The search strategy and decisions about inclusion and exclusion of studies should be shaped by the review questions. The PICO or SPICE frameworks for developing review questions (see p. 24) can be helpful in focusing the question(s) to facilitate searching. However, no matter how well-defined the review questions and scope, searching for studies can be very complex and time-consuming despite its seeming simplicity. The more broadly the review questions are set, the more time-consuming and complex the searching process will be. Ideally, reviewers should make time to develop and test the search strategy to ensure it is as comprehensive as time allows, but that it does not generate a large amount of what turns out to be irrelevant material. Getting expert help from an information scientist or librarian knowledgeable in the field is usually a worthwhile investment.

Once the precise review questions have been defined the preliminary search (see above) can be extended and/or refined. This may include further searching of electronic databases as well as other sources such as: internet searches using search engines such as Google Scholar, conference proceedings, abstracts of theses and dissertations, personal contact with researchers in the field, hand searching of specialist journals, published bibliographies and scanning of reference lists from previous reviews and individual studies already identified. It is just as important to keep a record of the search strategy and terms used for searching the internet and other sources as part of the audit trail or account of the review process as it is to document the searches of electronic bibliographic databases.

In most reviews, and particularly those intending to include qualitative research and other social science studies, the reviewers will have to search other sources besides electronic databases. For example, sometimes the 'grey' literature of unpublished reports will constitute the bulk of the evidence on a particular topic. Judgement needs to be exercised about how much relevant material is likely to be missed by electronic databases and the resources available for other forms of searching. In a review of the effectiveness of crime prevention interventions, for example, the authors obtained more than half their articles from reviewing reference lists and talking to contacts (Casteel and Peek-Asa 2000).

There have been major advances in the procedures used to search electronic databases for quantitative studies of effectiveness, especially in the health field, that maximise both comprehensiveness and precision (Dickersin et al. 1994; Glanville et al. 1998). However, the relationship between the comprehensiveness and precision of electronic search strategies becomes more problematic when the studies to be identified are more diverse in their focus and design (Shaw et al. 2004). Also in other areas of the social sciences, databases and the quality of abstracts are far less well developed for efficient searching. For this reason, reviewers need to be fully conversant with the subject in question to ensure that all relevant search terms are included and to avoid locating huge amounts of irrelevant material (Grayson and Gomersall 2003).

Searching for qualitative research using electronic databases can be particularly frustrating, although the problems encountered here can also be a feature of electronic searches for quantitative research other than on effectiveness. There are no equivalents to the Cochrane database of randomised trials for qualitative research. Poor indexing in databases and the diversity of qualitative research make the development of search strategies for identifying qualitative studies difficult. Some databases do not index qualitative studies at all – for example, PubMed only included the index term 'qualitative research' from 2003 whilst others (such as CINAHL) use a number of methodological indexing terms appropriate to qualitative study designs (Evans 2002a). The use of different databases will increase the coverage of different types of evidence, for example, OPAC will retrieve books and some book chapters. CINAHL has a particular focus on nursing and allied health-related research and is also reasonably helpful in locating theses and dissertations.

If the review is going to include a range of study designs, then electronic search terms should not generally involve study design or methodologic filters (sometimes referred to as 'hedges'). However if the search needs to focus on qualitative research, Grant (2004) suggests using the terms 'qualitative$', 'findings' and 'interview$' (where $ denotes truncation) as a way of identifying qualitative research designs. There are an increasing number of protocols designed to improve the accuracy (or relevance) of electronic searches for qualitative studies (such as from the Health Care Practice Research and Development Unit at the University of Salford, UK at http://www.fhsc.salford.ac.uk/hcprdu/projects/qualitative.htm). Similarly, others have adapted protocols designed specifically to search for qualitative studies in systematic reviews (Popay et al. 1998). However, research developing and testing different electronic search strategies to identify qualitative studies continues to highlight problems. For example, recent research evaluating the performance of three search strategies for qualitative research on breastfeeding using six electronic bibliographic databases (Shaw et al. 2004) reported that of 7420 records retrieved by the three strategies only 262 were relevant to the review. These findings suggest the need for considerable improvements in the way in which different qualitative research methods are described in journal abstracts and indexed in bibliographic databases.

For those wanting more advice on searching, Chapter 4 of Petticrew and Roberts (2006) is devoted entirely to searching and includes a wealth of sources, practical tips and general principles which there is not space to discuss here.

Inclusion criteria

For systematic reviews of effectiveness, formal hierarchies based on study design (see Box 1.4, p. 12) are often used to set inclusion and exclusion criteria, on the grounds that for the questions these reviews typically attempt to answer, the most important criterion of quality is the maximisation of internal validity (to ensure that like-with-like comparisons are made). One of the most sophisticated is the Oxford Centre for Evidence-Based Medicine's 'grading system for studies of prevention, diagnosis, prognosis, therapy and harm' (http://www.cebm.net/levels_of_evidence.asp).

There remains controversy over the assumptions inherent in these quality assessments and how they should be used to influence the overall interpretation of study findings since they are based on the design of studies. However, there is an acceptance that it is desirable and theoretically possible to use generalisable structured appraisal procedures to minimise error. It is also accepted that clear and transparent approaches for judging 'good' research are needed. However, even where clear criteria have been set – for example, the Consort statement on randomised controlled trials (Moher et al. 2001) spelling out how they should be conducted and reported – the information required to assess quality as opposed to basic design, is not always available in research reports. As a result, it can be difficult to distinguish in practice between a poorly designed and conducted RCT (ostensibly superior to other comparative experimental designs), and a well-designed and well-conducted prospective comparative cohort study which could well produce findings less susceptible to bias than the weak RCT.

Other approaches have few exclusion criteria, but exclude only 'fatally flawed' studies at a fairly early stage in the review process (but not necessarily before any data extraction and analysis has taken place).

Quality appraisal

The following section reviews some of the approaches to quality appraisal that might be used for synthesis. Quality appraisal is also called validity assessment, assessment of study quality or critical appraisal. It refers to the process of assessing the methodological quality of individual studies and may or may not be associated with decisions on which studies to include or exclude. The process of quality appraisal is important as the quality of studies or other evidence may affect both the results of the individual studies and ultimately the conclusions reached from the synthesis. However, 'quality' in general, and validity in particular are defined differently in relation to different types of study designs and research traditions (see earlier discussions about 'the hierarchy of evidence' p. 12).

In the context of an effectiveness review, study quality is primarily judged in terms of internal validity (i.e. to ensure that the study makes like-with-like comparisons), thus focusing on issues such as selection bias, drop-out rates, 'contamination' between cases and controls, and observer bias. There are many checklists available to assess the quality of quantitative studies along these lines (Chalmers et al. 1981; Downs and Black 1998; Jadad 1998; NHS Centre for Reviews and Dissemination 2001), but they should not be used slavishly, if only because all studies have weaknesses – the question is whether they matter and how much in the circumstances of the review. Some checklists invite the researcher to produce an overall 'score' for each study (e.g. trial), which can lead to excluding all studies that fall below a particular level. For example the Jadad (1998) scale is based on whether the study was randomised and double blinded, if there was a description of attrition and if the analysis was arrived out on an 'intention to treat' basis. The resulting score from this scale can be used to decide whether to include a study in a review. However, making an exclusion decision on the basis of such a score can be a risky approach because different aspects of study design and execution may be more or less important in specific reviews depending on the topic and question. It is preferable when making inclusion and exclusion decisions based on quality (if this is judged to be necessary) to decide what are likely to be the most important flaws in the context of the particular review, to read each study carefully and then to make a judgement on inclusion or not. Sometimes an otherwise weak study includes important information which can be used to help with the interpretation of findings from better studies and so is not excluded, but the reasons for retention are specified. For example, a weak effectiveness study might give valid information about how a particular intervention works.

For reviews incorporating qualitative research, the issue of quality appraisal is even more problematic. Here, the debate centres on two issues: whether the concepts of methodological quality used should be roughly the same as, or quite different from, those currently used to assess quantitative research and whether the judgement about quality should be made before or during the synthesis of findings from included studies. Some commentators take an extreme view and argue, for example, that quality cannot be judged against prescribed standards (Howe and Eisenhart 1990; Garratt and Hodkinson 1998). Others accept the need for more structured procedures and argue for standard criteria against which qualitative research may be assessed, but diverge between those who emphasise criteria familiar to quantitative researchers such as inter-observer reliability and construct validity, and those who emphasise more subjective criteria such as authenticity and credibility of accounts (Lincoln and Guba 1985; Seale and Silverman 1997; Attree and Milton 2006). In the health field, the UK NHS Centre for Reviews and Dissemination (CRD) favours a priori structured quality assessment of qualitative studies for inclusion in reviews, but recognises that a vast number of different schemata exist for assessing quality of qualitative studies (NHS CRD 2001; Spencer et al. 2003). Elsewhere, some approaches, such as meta-ethnography, take the view that the worth of particular studies may become apparent only during the synthesis process (Noblit and Hare 1988) and syntheses have incorporated studies regarded as weak (c.f. Campbell et al. 2003).

Suffice it to say that, whilst it is important that reviewers have some sense of the rigour of the studies included and take account of this in some way during the synthesis, the presence of multiple, different checklists (see the useful review of these by Spencer et al. 2003), the lack of agreement about which quality criteria to use, how cut off points are to be applied, and whether to exclude studies judged to be methodologically weak, make it difficult to prescribe a single approach to the assessment of quality in qualitative research or synthesis. At present the most useful quality appraisal frameworks for qualitative research appear to be those developed by Spencer et al. 2003 (see Box 2.2) and the Critical Appraisal Tool for qualitative research studies developed by the Public Health Resource Unit at the University of Salford http://www.phru.nhs.uk/casp/critical_appraisal_tools.htm#qualitative.

The CASP tool has been adapted and used in synthesis of qualitative research (Pound et al. 2005). In addition the Joanna Briggs Institute has developed an appraisal tool for assessing qualitative research (Qualitative Assessment and Review Instrument (JBI-QARI)) as part of its software to support reviews (see: http://www.joannabriggs.edu.au/services/sumari.php).

Box 2.2 Example of a quality appraisal framework (Spencer et al. 2003)	
a) Appraisal questions	**b) Quality indicators (possible features for consideration)**
How credible are the findings?	Findings/conclusions are supported by data/study evidence *(i.e. the reader can see how the researcher arrived at his/her conclusions; the 'buildings blocks' of analysis and interpretation are evident)*
	Findings/conclusions 'make sense'/have a coherent logic
	Findings/conclusions are resonant with other knowledge and experience *(this might include peer or member review)*
	Use of corroborating evidence to support or refine findings (i.e. other data sources have been used to examine phenomena; other research evidence has been evaluated: see also Q14)
How has knowledge/ understanding been extended by the research?	Literature review (where appropriate) summarising knowledge to date/key issues raised by previous research
	Aims and design of study set in the context of existing knowledge/understanding; identifies new areas for investigation *(for example, in relation to policy/practice/substantive theory)*
	Credible/clear discussion of how findings have contributed to knowledge and understanding *(e.g. of the policy, programme or theory being reviewed)*; might be applied to new policy developments, practice or theory
	Findings presented or conceptualised in a way that offers new insights/alternative ways of thinking
	Discussion of limitations of evidence and what remains unknown/unclear or what further information/research is needed
How well does the evaluation address its original aims and purpose?	Clear statement of study aims and objectives; reasons for any changes in objectives
	Findings clearly linked to the purposes of the study – and to the initiative or policy being studied

	Summary or conclusions directed towards aims of study
	Discussion of limitations of study in meeting aims *(e.g. are there limitations because of restricted access to study settings or participants, gaps in the sample coverage, missed or unresolved areas of questioning: incomplete analysis: time constraints?)*
Scope for drawing wider inference – how well is this explained?	Discussion of what can be generalised to wider population from which sample is drawn/case selection has been made
	Detailed description of the contexts in which the study was conducted to allow applicability to other settings/contextual generalities to be assessed
	Discussion of how hypotheses/propositions/ findings may relate to wider theory; consideration of rival explanations
	Evidence supplied to support claims for wider inference *(either from study or from corroborating sources)*
	Discussion of limitations on drawing wider inference *(e.g. re-examination of sample and any missing constituencies: analysis of restrictions of study settings for drawing wider inference)*
How clear is the basis of evaluative appraisal?	Discussion of how assessments of effectiveness/evaluative judgements have been reached *(i.e. whose judgements are they and on what basis have they been reached?)*
	Description of any formalised appraisal criteria used; when generated and how and by whom they have been applied
	Discussion of the nature and source of any divergence in evaluative appraisals
	Discussion of any unintended consequences of intervention, their impact and why they arose
How defensible is the research design?	Discussion of how overall research strategy was designed to meet aims of study
	Discussion of rationale for study design

(continued overleaf)

Box 2.2 (continued)	
	Convincing argument for different features of research design *(e.g. reasons given for different components or stages of research; purpose of particular methods or data sources, multiple methods, time frames etc.)*
	Use of different features of design/data sources evident in findings presented
	Discussion of limitations of research design and their implications for the study evidence
How well defended is the sample design/target selection of cases/documents?	Description of study locations/areas and how and why chosen
	Description of population of interest and how sample selection relates to it *(e.g. typical, extreme case, diverse constituencies etc.)*
	Rationale for basis of selection of target sample/settings/documents *(e.g. characteristics/ features of target sample/settings/documents, basis for inclusions and exclusions, discussion of sample size/number of cases/setting selected etc)*
	Discussion of how sample/selections allowed required comparisons to be made
Sample composition/case inclusion – how well is the eventual coverage described?	Detailed profile of achieved sample/case coverage
	Maximising inclusion *(e g language matching or translation; specialised recruitment; organised transport for group attendance)*
	Discussion of any missing coverage in achieved samples/cases and implications for study evidence *(e.g. through comparison of target and achieved samples, comparison with population etc.)*
	Documentation of reasons for non-participation among sample approached/non-inclusion of selected cases/documents
	Discussion of access and methods of approach and how these might have affected participation/coverage

How well was the data collection carried out?	Discussion of:
	• procedures/documents used for collection/ recording
	• who conducted data collection
	• checks on origin/status/authorship of documents
	Audio or video recording of interviews/discussions/ conversations *(if not recorded, were justifiable reasons given?)*
	Description of conventions for taking fieldnotes *(e.g. to identify what form of observations were required/to distinguish description from researcher commentary/analysis)*
	Discussion of how fieldwork methods or settings may have influenced data collected
	Demonstration, through portrayal and use of data, that depth, detail and richness were achieved in collection
How well has the approach to, and formulation of, the analysis been conveyed?	Description of form of original data *(e.g. use of verbatim transcripts, observation or interview notes, documents, etc.)*
	Clear rationale for choice of data management method/tool/package
	Evidence of how <u>descriptive</u> analytic categories, classes, labels etc. have been generated and used *(i.e. either through explicit discussion or portrayal in the commentary)*
	Discussion, with examples, of how any <u>constructed</u> analytic concepts/typologies etc. have been devised and applied
Contexts of data sources – how well are they retained and portrayed?	Description of background or historical developments and social/organisational characteristics of study sites or settings
	Participants' perspectives/observations placed in personal context *(e.g. use of case studies/vignettes/ individual profiles, textual extracts annotated with details of contributors)*

(continued overleaf)

Box 2.2 (continued)	
	Explanation of origins/history of written documents
	Use of data management methods that preserve context *(i.e. facilitate within case description and analysis)*
How well has diversity of perspective and content been explored?	Discussion of contribution of sample design/case selection in generating diversity
	Description and illumination of diversity/multiple perspectives/alternative positions in the evidence displayed
	Evidence of attention to negative cases, outliers or exceptions
	Typologies/models of variation derived and discussed
	Examination of origins/influences on opposing or differing positions
	Identification of patterns of association/linkages with divergent positions/groups
How well has detail, depth and complexity (i.e. richness) of the data been conveyed?	Use and exploration of contributors' terms, concepts and meanings
	Unpacking and portrayal of nuance/subtlety/intricacy within data
	Discussion of explicit and implicit explanations
	Detection of underlying factors/influences
	Identification and discussion of patterns of association/conceptual linkages within data
	Presentation of illuminating textual extracts/observations
How clear are the links between data, interpretation and conclusions – i.e. how well can the route to any conclusions be seen?	Clear conceptual links between analytic commentary and presentations of original data *(i.e. commentary and cited data relate; there is an analytic context to cited data, not simply repeated description)*
	Discussion of how/why particular interpretation/significance is assigned to specific aspects of data – with illustrative extracts of original data

	Discussion of how explanations/ theories/ conclusions were derived – and how they relate to interpretations and content of original data (*i.e. how warranted*); whether alternative explanations explored
	Display of negative cases and how they lie outside main proposition/theory/ hypothesis etc.; or how proposition etc. revised to include them
How clear and coherent is the reporting?	Demonstrates link to aims of study/research questions
	Provides a narrative/story or clearly constructed thematic account
	Has structure and signposting that usefully guide reader through the commentary
	Provides accessible information for intended target audience(s)
	Key messages highlighted or summarised
How clear are the assumptions/ theoretical perspectives/values that have shaped the form and output of the evaluation?	Discussion/evidence of the main assumptions/ hypotheses/theoretical ideas on which the evaluation was based and how these affected the form, coverage or output of the evaluation (*the assumption here is that no research is undertaken without some underlying assumptions or theoretical ideas*)
	Discussion/evidence of the ideological perspectives/values/philosophies of research team and their impact on the methodological or substantive content of the evaluation (*again, may not be explicitly stated*)
	Evidence of openness to new/alternative ways of viewing subject/theories/ assumptions (*e.g. discussion of learning/concepts/constructions that have emerged from the data; refinement restatement of hypotheses/theories in light of emergent findings; evidence that alternative claims have been examined*)
	Discussion of how error or bias may have arisen in design/data collection/analysis and how addressed, if at all
	Reflections on the impact of the researcher on the research process

(continued overleaf)

Box 2.2 (continued)	
What evidence is there of attention to ethical issues?	Evidence of thoughtfulness/sensitivity about research contexts and participants
	Documentation of how research was presented in study settings/to participants *(including, where relevant, any possible consequences of taking part)*
	Documentation of consent procedures and information provided to participants
	Discussion of confidentiality of data and procedures for protecting
	Discussion of how anonymity of participants/ sources was protected
	Discussion of any measures to offer information/ advice/services etc. at end of study *(i.e. where participation exposed the need for these)*
	Discussion of potential harm or difficulty through participation, and how avoided
How adequately has the research process been documented?	Discussion of strengths and weaknesses of data sources and methods
	Documentation of changes made to design and reasons; implications for study coverage
	Documentation and reasons for changes in sample coverage/data collection/analytic approach; implications
	Reproduction of main study documents *(e.g. letters of approach, topic guides, observation templates, data management frameworks etc.,)*

Given the discussion thus far it will be clear that for reviews that attempt to include diverse evidence the issue of quality selection is highly problematic. While much of the discussion here has focused on the assessment of quality in research, the reviewer must address similar issues in relation to any non-research sources of evidence to be included.

Approaches to quality appraisal of diverse evidence can be divided into two, depending on whether they propose quantitative criteria (which allow for a cut-off point to be calculated, and thus the exclusion of studies – see above for a discussion of the pitfalls of scoring and quantitative cut-offs) or qualitative criteria without scores. According to Murphy et al. (1998), validity and relevance are the underlying criteria which unify seemingly quite distinct approaches. Additionally, as Brannen (1992) notes, there are considerable overlaps between the general quality criteria used in relation to both qualitative and quantitative research, although there are important differences in how they may be interpreted and applied. The problem facing those wishing to use such criteria to assess qualitative and quantitative research for synthesis is determining which approaches should be used and how the criteria should be applied. Some use quality appraisal as a moderator – to facilitate decisions about inclusion and exclusion on the basis of the weight or worth of a particular piece of evidence. Others use such frameworks to provide a series of prompts or points for consideration during the review process. Most qualitative assessment frameworks tend not to specify how judgements should be made on whether or not a standard has been reached (Harden and Thomas 2005) and typically do not indicate how much weight should be given to evidence from studies of different quality. The JBI-QARI software currently being developed does allow specific weighting of the credibility of studies in a review, but it remains to be seen whether researchers will use this facility, and if they do, whether they will find it helpful.

Whatever approach is taken, there is a need for careful records to be kept about the appraisal process (which should ideally involve at least two researchers) ensuring that both the strengths and weaknesses of the research and other sources are recorded so that this information can be used appropriately in a later stage of the review when the findings are being synthesized and interpreted, as well as by readers of the review.

Data extraction

Data extraction is often described as if it follows the assessment of study quality and the application of inclusion and exclusion criteria, but, of course, in practice, it is virtually impossible to make decisions about whether a study is within the scope of the review question or of sufficient quality without a good knowledge of study content and this is difficult to do consistently across a number of studies without extracting information from the text reporting each study in a consistent way. So data extraction is usually part of the previous two elements of a review.

Decisions about which data should be extracted from individual studies should be guided primarily by the review question(s). In the context of a systematic review of the effectiveness of a particular intervention, for example, the data to be extracted should include details of: the participants; the interventions; the comparisons; the outcomes; and, where used, the study design. The other information to be extracted is usually that which could affect the interpretation of the study results or that which might be helpful in assessing how applicable the results were to different population groups or other settings. For example, if there are reasons to believe that the intervention will produce different effects across various age or other social groups, then it is important to extract information relevant to the subgroups of interest. Similarly, it is important to extract information about the setting in which the intervention takes place, particularly if the review is addressing questions about implementation. For example, in the case of interventions to prevent unintentional injury, the settings might include home and school or different types of neighbourhood. The intervention should also be described, particularly if there is interest in which elements of the intervention are most important in producing its effects. This would involve extracting data about the content, format and timing of the intervention, who was involved in delivering it, how it was delivered and so on.

For reviews of quantitative studies, outcome data are best recorded, at least initially, as presented in the original paper (e.g. as means and standard deviations or odds ratios and confidence intervals), or in a form that will allow effect sizes to be calculated. Outcome data would not normally be transformed into a common form at this stage – this would be done, if appropriate, before or during the synthesis stage. Where study design is used as a key criterion of quality the design features of each study should also be described.

When looking at qualitative studies or more mixed sources of evidence, the data extraction process may be more complex. Initially it can be useful to build up a summary of each of the individual studies, as in a systematic review of effectiveness, for example, noting the study design and methods used, the number and characteristics of participants and the setting or context. Where the material to be synthesized is mainly qualitative, the data extraction is likely to be dependent on the synthesis method chosen (see Chapters 4 and 5), but broadly a way needs to be found to capture the findings of interest. For example in an interpretive synthesis (see Chapter 4), this will be the interpretations offered by the authors, typically in the form of analytical concepts, metaphors or themes, but in a realist synthesis (see Chapter 5), the focus will be less on specific concepts and more on overarching theories or explanations which can be synthesized.

The way data are extracted and stored varies among reviewers. There are various computer software programmes that can support this process, ranging from the simple (for example commonly used spreadsheets and databases such as MS Excel and MS Access) to those specifically designed for this purpose such as RevMan and SUMARI. Chapters 4 and 6 both detail some of the different ways of displaying data to facilitate comparisons in a synthesis and many of the basic matrix or charting approaches can also be used for data extraction. Whichever method is chosen, it is worth creating a standard record of the data extracted as this can enable sharing of the material within teams of reviewers, and in the long term provides a transparent record of how this part of the review was undertaken.

Synthesis

Synthesis is the point in the review process at which the findings from the included studies are combined in order to draw conclusions based on the studies as a whole. Chapters 3–5 describe different methods for synthesis that have potential application to diverse sources of evidence. As already noted, reviews designed to support policy and management decision-making are likely to include heterogeneous sources and forms of evidence, and will typically have to adopt a broadly narrative based approach to synthesis – in essence they will need to tell a story summarising the body of evidence synthesized in the review. There are also more specialised methods for synthesizing particular kinds of research, such as meta-ethnography in relation to qualitative research, and statistical meta-analysis for some kinds of homogeneous quantitative evidence such as RCTs. Occasionally an entire review will be based on one of these specialised synthesis techniques, but it is perfectly appropriate for a review to incorporate a number of different syntheses of different types of evidence linked together by an overarching narrative (see Chapters 5 and 8 for more on combining different synthesis methods in a single review).

Specific methods for synthesis are discussed in more detail later in the book in the relevant chapters, but in summary the process entails organising the relevant evidence extracted from the included sources and then finding some way of bringing it together. The way the evidence is organised depends to some extent on the type(s) and scope of evidence, the method(s) employed and on the preferences of the reviewer. As with data extraction, the process of organising the studies is often facilitated by the use of charts or tables summarising key aspects of the studies. The format of these is largely dependent on how many studies or pieces of evidence are included, but these need to be capable of allowing repeated examination and comparison of the relevant data from each study. An obvious approach is to compare the findings of studies on the basis of study design and study quality. For quantitative synthesis, charts will need to summarise or present statistical or numerical information whereas for qualitative and mixed forms of evidence the materials displayed are likely to be textual summaries and/or themes.

For interpretive (Chapter 4) and mixed (Chapter 5) syntheses it can also be helpful to organise the evidence into thematic or conceptual groupings. In meta-ethnography, for example, one of the included papers is often used as an 'index' paper as a way of orienting the synthesis. This may be a classic or perhaps the earliest paper on the topic which provides a starting point for the synthesis process. In addition, it may be necessary to further sub-divide the material to be synthesized into more manageable groupings. For example, in their meta-ethnography of 37 papers on medicine-taking, Pound et al. (2005) grouped the papers into medicine groups and synthesized the findings within these groups before looking across all the studies. Greenhalgh et al. (2005) chose to organise the large and complex literature on innovations described in Chapter 1 (see p. 7) into broad disciplinary groupings (e.g. from rural sociology, evidence-based medicine) and then to plot their contributions chronologically in order to map the development of theory and evidence in this area.

Chapters 3–5 of this book discuss specific approaches to synthesis most likely to be relevant to reviews of diverse evidence. Chapter 6 describes in more detail a range of different ways of organising data for synthesis and subsequent presentation. A useful source of further reading is also the chapter by Petticrew and Roberts (2006: 164–214) which provides a more general overview of the steps involved in synthesis with helpful examples.

Writing up and dissemination

It is self-evident that for research or reviews to be useful, they need to be comprehensible and accessible. This means that findings need to be communicated effectively. However, the key to effective implementation in policy and practice lies in both appropriate reporting and dissemination of results, and in understanding that reporting and dissemination alone are not enough. Much is known about how to produce accessible reports and how to disseminate these effectively, but less is known about how effective implementation is achieved. These issues and more detailed guidance where it is available are discussed in Part 3 of this book.

PART 2
Methods for evidence synthesis

The synthesis of diverse sources of evidence may be an emerging area of research but there are already a number of apparently different methods for synthesis available. Dixon-Woods et al. (2005) outlined some eleven possible approaches to syntheses involving qualitative and quantitative evidence, and there are yet more methods described in the methods literature. Some of the apparent diversity of method can be attributed to the differential labelling of what are in essence the same methods; some is linked to the inevitable process of adapting methods in practice and also to the temptation facing authors to re-badge techniques as a way of staking a claim to a particular approach. Notwithstanding this, synthesis is a rapidly developing area of research methodology and one in which new techniques are likely to emerge in the future.

Rather than attempt to outline all the possible methods currently available for synthesis, this book focuses on three broad approaches to the challenges of synthesizing diverse evidence sources and illustrates each with examples of specific techniques which have potential application to synthesis for policy- and decision-making. Chapter 3 describes synthesis approaches which are broadly quantitative; in essence, these entail transforming evidence into numbers, to enable relatively simple counts or more sophisticated statistical or logical analyses. Chapter 4 provides information about the qualitative counterparts to these quantitative approaches and looks at methods that use text based data or transform other evidence into this form. Importantly, however, it only focuses on approaches that are interpretive. These approaches use comparative or translational synthesis methods to generate conceptual and theoretical interpretations or explanations of a body of evidence drawn from different sources. Developed from the interpretive paradigm within social science research, these methods have largely been employed for the synthesis of qualitative research alone, rather than in conjunction with quantitative evidence. Nonetheless they have the potential to be used in reviews that include more diverse evidence. The closing chapter of Part 2, Chapter 5, looks at a number of other approaches to evidence review and synthesis that do not 'fit' readily into either the quantitative or interpretive categories of the two preceding chapters. The approaches documented in this chapter are characterised by their eclecticism, drawing on text-based (qualitative) and quantitative methods for synthesis, sometimes in parallel, sometimes in sequence. Compared to the synthesis methods described in Chapters 3 and 4, the methods in Chapter 5 engage, in very different ways, with the challenge of synthesizing diverse forms of evidence to inform policy and management decision-making.

3 Quantitative approaches to evidence synthesis

The quantitative synthesis methods included in this chapter have potential for handling complex bodies of evidence: whether qualitative or quantitative. Although some of these methods were devised for primary research, they all have potential application to the synthesis of findings from existing studies. They all involve the conversion of data (whether qualitative or quantitative) into quantitative (i.e. numerical) form for simple counts and more sophisticated statistical analyses, and for use in logical (Boolean) analysis. This entails transforming qualitative findings into numbers by identifying themes which can then become variables that can be quantified either as frequency counts or in binary form. This is controversial as Petticrew and Roberts (2006: 191) point out:

> Perhaps the least useful way of dealing with qualitative data in systematic reviews is to turn it [*sic*] into quantitative data. While it would make the job of systematizing qualitative research easy if it were restricted to 'x participants in y studies said z', this is unlikely to be helpful and is a waste of the qualitative data. If one wishes to know how many people say 'z', then a well-designed survey is likely to be the method of choice.

This warning is a wise one and care should be taken with the methods described in this chapter. Before attempting to integrate findings from qualitative and quantitative studies or from multiple qualitative studies into some quantitative form, one should always consider whether two separate syntheses with an overall narrative commentary would work better and represent the original findings more faithfully, or even whether original research would be better than a review. Often, however, undertaking comparable original research is not feasible, for example, if one wants to extract generalisable understanding from events that occurred at different times in the past (e.g. undertaking a synthesis of studies of major health care system reforms in order to try to tease out the factors associated with more and less 'successful' changes).

As noted earlier, reviews of topics and questions of significance for policy-makers and other decision-makers will often have to grapple with complex bodies of evidence so simply reporting findings from parallel syntheses of qualitative and quantitative studies may be both ponderous and a recipe for making inadequate use of both sources. There have been a number of methodological innovations in recent years designed to enable qualitative findings to be used in the synthesis of quantitative evidence. Perhaps the most notable efforts have been Bayesian approaches to meta-analysis and the linking of systematic reviews that include meta-analyses to decision analyses. These are discussed below. This chapter also describes techniques designed less to synthesize qualitative and quantitative evidence than to enable predominantly qualitative studies to be synthesized in a quantitative way with the aim of establishing valid generalisations across individual qualitative case studies. In particular, it describes 'qualitative comparative analysis' (Ragin 1987) which is a method for analysing and making overall sense of multiple case studies (these could include both qualitative and quantitative evidence) using Boolean algebra. This method is discussed at the end of this chapter, but the chapter opens with a description of the more straightforward technique of content analysis.

Content analysis

What is it?

Content analysis was developed for primary research on a wide variety of mainly textual information (Hodson 1999a) but it can be used to synthesize findings from published research studies to identify dominant findings and, thereby, make generalisations. As an approach to synthesis of existing research, at its simplest, it provides a systematic technique for categorising data from different studies into themes (categories) and then counting how often each theme occurs. Quantitative content analysis measures frequencies and this distinguishes this method from 'thematic analysis' and qualitative forms of content analysis which are used to analyse and group concepts and themes, but do not attempt to count them (see Chapter 5 for a discussion of these approaches). Like the 'quantitative case survey' described below, content analysis uses a standard data extraction instrument (i.e. a questionnaire) to aid the reproducibility of the data collection and coding. The text of both qualitative and quantitative studies can be synthesized using content analysis, depending on the synthesis question. Content analysis can also be used with visual materials such as video recordings, photographs or artwork.

According to Stemler (2001), content analysis is defined as 'a systematic, replicable technique for compressing many words of text into fewer content categories based on explicit rules of coding'. Bryman (2004: 181) has a broader definition: 'Content analysis is an approach to the analysis of documents and texts (which may be printed or visual), that seeks to quantify content in terms of predetermined categories and in a systematic and replicable manner.' Both these definitions view content analysis as essentially a quantitative method since all the data are eventually converted into frequencies, though qualitative skills and an understanding of underlying theory may be needed to develop the themes or categories into which findings are to be fitted, and to identify the relationship(s) between the raw data and particular categories or themes.

In order to undertake content analysis the categories of interest have to be defined sufficiently precisely in advance for multiple assessors to be able to code the same data in the same way (e.g. a transcript of a television interview). As a result, categories must be exclusive and exhaustive. Examples of the kinds of thing that can be identified and counted include: the identity of the person speaking or writing; the subject matter; conflicts of view; the specific words used to describe something; the disposition of the speaker or writer (i.e. for or against a proposition) and so on.

In the context of reviews of qualitative and quantitative research for policy and management, content analysis may be useful in presenting a quantitative picture derived from a range of qualitative and quantitative information. This would have to be undertaken with care since, for example, the number of times a concept is mentioned in the report of a qualitative study partly depends on the extent to which the report comprises quotes from participants (who may not use the particular conceptual term at all) versus the researchers' interpretation and discussion of what participants were saying. Despite this, content analysis has potential utility, for example, in assessing the likely acceptability of a range of different policy solutions to a problem by determining the degree of media support over time for each solution and the most frequently voiced public criticisms in the media. This understanding could then be used in the development and implementation of a new, improved intervention for the problem in question. An example of a content analysis of change in media coverage of a policy issue over time is given in Miller and Reilly's (1995) account of British newspaper coverage of so-called 'food scares', especially salmonella in eggs and other foods. They found that coverage had more or less disappeared after an initial peak just as the incidence of salmonella poisoning was rising. This suggests that the level of media coverage is a poor indicator of the impact of a problem on the community compared to its salience in the hierarchy of popular concerns.

There are relatively few examples of syntheses based on content analysis. However, Hodson (1999b) cited in Bryman (2004: 196), used content analysis explicitly as a method to synthesize a set of mainly qualitative studies. Hodson synthesized 106 published, detailed, ethnographic case studies from a number of countries of job satisfaction and worker autonomy in different types of workplace in order to look at the effect of type of workplace on the workers. A theoretically informed coding structure was developed so that each workplace was coded into one of five types: craft; direct supervision; assembly line; bureaucratic; and worker participation. Job satisfaction was coded from 1 = very low to 5 = very high and worker autonomy from 1 = none (the workers' tasks are completely determined by others, by machines or by organisational rules) to 5 = very high (significant interpretation is needed to reach broadly specified goals). Hodson found that some of the more pessimistic accounts of worker participation schemes (e.g. those that concluded that they did not allow genuine participation or that they did not have a positive effect on workers' job satisfaction) were empirically incomplete when viewed from the perspective of the more positive studies.

What are the strengths and limitations of content analysis?

Content analysis has the advantage of being well developed and widely used (e.g. most notably in media studies, especially of political bias in news reporting). Unlike many of the methods for synthesis discussed in this book it is also a technique that has been developed for the analysis of published or broadcast texts and materials rather than primary research data, and this may make it especially useful in the synthesis of a variety of published forms of evidence (e.g. research papers, government reports, news media) for policy- and decision-making since these are already in text form.

Various computer software packages are available to support content analyses (see Box 3.1). These make it possible to handle large amounts of text straightforwardly and systematically in a short space of time. Content analysis is a flexible technique since it can be applied to a large range of different kinds of structured and unstructured information, and the steps in content analysis can be easily described making it transparent and reproducible. The results are also relatively easy and economical to present, consisting of tabulations of frequency counts and they can be fed into a variety of statistical analyses.

However, content analysis can be criticised for being too reductive and for emphasising those phenomena that are amenable to being counted rather than those that are significant interpretively. For instance, while content analysis is a good means of determining how often a politician makes reference to a particular thinker, it cannot so easily be used to identify the importance of that thinker in shaping the politician's own thinking or why the politician is particularly attracted to the particular thinker's ideas. Though coding in content analysis can be developed so that it becomes far more sophisticated than simple counts of the use of individual words (e.g. coding can be devised to capture the simultaneous expression of a group of related ideas), it is essentially a technique for simplifying phenomena since it reduces large amounts of data (e.g. text and speech) into a relatively small number of categories.

Box 3.1   Quantitative software for content analysis

Wordsmith – This is one of the Wordsmith Tools developed by Mick Scott, and available under licence. It enables the development of word lists and clusters, and allows the user to view where in the original document/text each occurrence comes, as well as allowing statistical analyses. It can be used for a range of different languages. http://www.lexically.net/wordsmith/index.html

Textpack – This is a system for computer-aided quantitative content analysis designed for exploring and editing texts. It enables the categorisation of texts against analytic dictionaries which can be developed and validated using the software. Numeric output is compatible with statistical packages like SPSS or SAS. It can be used for English or Spanish language texts. http://www.gesis.org/en/software/textpack/

TACT – Text Analysis Computing Tools. A text analysis and retrieval system, with 15 separate programs, it was designed for use in literary studies. It runs within MS-DOS and can sort frequencies of words or phrases and perform rankings. It can be used in English, French, German, Italian, Spanish, Latin, and other modern European languages or languages using a roman alphabet, and classical Greek. http://www.chass.utoronto.ca/tact/index.html

Textstat – is a simple text analysis tool developed by the Dutch Linguistics group at the Free University of Berlin. It is especially useful for the analysis of web based materials. It can read ASCII/ANSI texts and HTML files (directly from the internet) to produce word frequency lists. http://www.niederlandistik.fu-berlin.de/textstat/software-en.html

SPSS Text Analysis for Surveys – is a module within SPSS for coding and analysing open-ended survey questions. It can support text management, searching and textual analysis. It can be used to identify word stems and to automatically cluster terms that tend to occur together to create categories. It uses natural language processing text analysis to automate some of these processes and user-created categories can be developed. http://www.spss.com/textanalysis_surveys/capabilities.htm

---

Quantitative case survey

What is it?

The empirical literature in many fields of public policy tends to comprise a series of discrete case studies, making it difficult to generalise from the studies as a whole. The 'quantitative case survey' is one response to this limitation of case studies allowing statistical comparisons across studies. Essentially, the content of a series of case studies is extracted for analysis using a structured questionnaire so that comparable data can be collected from each, thereby allowing aggregation of findings and the identification of patterns in the data across case studies. It is thus a formal process for systematically coding data when there is a large enough number of independently conducted qualitative or mixed method studies to allow for subsequent quantitative analysis (Yin and Heald 1975; Larsson 1993). A questionnaire consisting of a set of structured, closed questions is used to extract data from individual case studies which are then treated as observations within a single quantitative dataset. An example of the kinds of variable derived from this approach is provided by Yin and Yates (1975; see Box 3.2). The quality of each case study can also be assessed based on the data extracted and certain studies may be excluded on grounds of either internal (potential for bias) or external (generalisability) validity.

After data extraction, the resulting dataset can then be used to construct cross-case matrices or summary tables in which each case study is summarised in terms of variables such as setting, the type of intervention, the design of the case study, the outcomes assessed, numbers of 'cases' and 'controls', if relevant, key findings, aspects of methodological quality, etc. The body of the table may simply record the presence or absence of a factor or the strength of an association or finding (e.g. the effect size of a programme), but it can include a summary of the data (e.g. the numbers of cases and controls in an experimental design). These matrices and summary tables are similar to comparative summary tables used in other approaches to synthesis (see Chapter 4, pp. 88–9).

The quantitative case survey method allows the more ambitious analyst to

---

Box 3.2 Example of quantitative case survey – the effectiveness of seven strategies of urban public service decentralisation (Yin and Yates 1975)

The following variables were extracted from each case study of decentralisation using a replicable approach, thereby allowing inter-analyst agreement to be measured between two researchers:

- research design and methods;
- background and context for the decentralisation initiative;
- characteristics of the decentralisation initiative (e.g. type of citizen participation, type of service involved, what was decentralised);
- outcomes of initiatives (improved information flow, improved staff attitudes to clients, improved client attitudes, improved services and increased client control or not).

go further and to convert data into quantitative form for statistical analysis of the associations between the outcome(s) of interest and various potentially explanatory variables across the case studies. If the case studies are sufficiently homogeneous this analysis could comprise a meta-analysis or other quantitative techniques (Cooper and Hedges 1994). Thus the case survey can be used as a way of turning what may be predominantly qualitative studies into quantitative data for analysis, thereby allowing an integrated qualitative–quantitative synthesis to be undertaken. Alternately it can be used as a technique to synthesize studies that are mainly quantitative as in the example of a quantitative case survey taken from Yin (1986) in Box 3.3. If there are too few studies for

---

Box 3.3   Example of case survey of evaluations of community crime prevention (Yin 1986)

Eleven evaluations of 11 different forms of crime prevention programme previously conducted by different investigators using a variety of mostly quantitative methods were dissected and compared to identify generalisable features of successful programmes which were independent of any specific form of intervention. All 11 evaluations had been deliberately chosen because they showed positive results despite each focusing on a different type of programme.

The aim was to enable policy-makers and programme managers to specify the minimum essential characteristics that all future programmes should exhibit to increase their likelihood of success.

The synthesis showed that the programmes were not unique (i.e. they could be repeated elsewhere); they had positive effects and the evaluations were robust and credible; they did not consistently target areas with the worst crime problems; they were probably not representative of all crime prevention programmes and evaluations; and useful but complex lessons for the US in the 1980s could be derived from the case studies, as follows:

- Crime prevention programmes taken singly rather than as part of a multi-faceted plan were likely to be ineffective;
- It was important to improve resident-police relationships and joint activities as part of any plan to prevent crime;
- Communities with the highest levels of crime were also likely to be those whose resident-police relationships were most difficult to improve except over a long period of time and at very considerable cost;
- As a result, it might not be possible to do much to prevent crime in the immediate future because the highest need areas were likely to be the most resistant to crime prevention initiatives.

quantitative analysis, the method can be used more simply to create text matrices and summary tables incorporating quantitative findings and text summaries. From this, it can be seen that the approach has much in common with content analysis as a method of synthesis.

The quantitative case survey method has also been used in primary research. The national evaluation of general practitioner 'total purchasing pilots' in the English NHS looked at the costs and benefits of allocating part of the NHS budget for specialist health services to general medical practices or groups of practices to enable them to purchase services for their enrolled patients (Goodwin et al. 1998). The researchers collected largely qualitative data from the 52 pilot sites. In addition to a qualitative thematic analysis, a closed questionnaire was used by three members of the research team to make a quantitative assessment of the degree to which each pilot had succeeded in bringing about desired local service change through its purchasing. This enabled agreed summary 'scores' to be produced representing each pilot's extent of achievement (see Figure 3.1). The scores were examined against a range of characteristics for each site extracted from interview data and other sources of data in a quantitative analysis. This analysis showed that the organisational type and the population size of each GP grouping were significantly correlated with the level of achievement.

What are the strengths and limitations of quantitative case surveys?

The case survey approach has the obvious advantage that it was specifically designed to handle multiple case studies. It allows the aggregation of findings

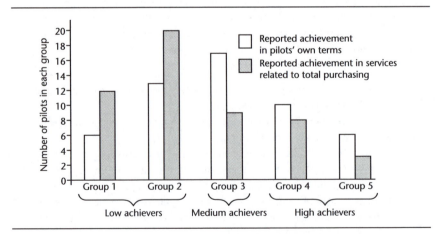

Figure 3.1   Total purchasing pilots by level of achievement (Goodwin et al. 1998)

across a series of studies of the same phenomenon. When there are large numbers of case studies, quantitative techniques can easily be used, including meta-analysis. Yin and Heald (1975) suggest that the method is particularly useful for synthesizing evidence on the impact of national social programmes that are implemented slightly differently between jurisdictions. The case survey method also lends itself to data extraction by multiple analysts, enabling the findings to be assessed for inter-rater reliability. This is a form of quality assurance that adds transparency to the approach – something that managers and policy-makers appear to value relatively highly in reviews (Martin 2005: 49). However, case survey is argued to be reductive by some qualitative researchers, despite the fact that characteristics such as the context of each case can be extracted and coded for use as explanatory variables. There is always a trade-off between the ability to generalise and the ability to understand fully all the nuances of individual cases.

The Bayesian approach

What is it?

Bayesian thinking offers one of the most attractive means for quantitative analysts to incorporate qualitative research data and other evidence into syntheses and analytical models designed to assist in policy and management decisions. In this group of methods, all data are converted into quantitative form, and pooled for analysis and modelling using Bayesian statistical methods. Bayesian approaches to synthesis are designed primarily to provide decision support (see Chapter 1, p. 14) and, accordingly, allow the incorporation of a wide range of evidence, including findings from qualitative research and subjective judgements (e.g. population or decision-makers' preferences and the trade-offs they are willing to make between policy goals derived from consensus methods (Black et al. 1999), in a quantitative synthesis.

A Bayesian approach can be used in a number of different types of synthesis where different forms of evidence need to be brought together, including cross-design synthesis (also known as 'grouped meta-analysis'), Bayesian meta-analysis, and comprehensive decision modelling or decision analysis. Cost-effectiveness analysis also lends itself to a Bayesian approach. Health economists are increasingly turning to Bayesian methods, particularly when cost-effectiveness analysis is to be used directly as an input to a specific decision, and also for sensitivity analysis. These different 'applications' of a Bayesian approach are briefly described below, but first it is worth outlining the key components of a Bayesian approach.

Applying Bayesian theory to synthesis

The basic idea behind Bayesian methods can be described in the following way. If a conventional clinical trial were carried out to find out by how much a new intervention A was superior or inferior to an existing intervention B for the same condition, the statistical analysis would yield, as summary results, a *P*-value, an estimate of effect and a confidence interval around the estimate. Bayesian analysis would supplement this by focusing not just on the question 'what is the effect of intervention A versus intervention B?', but further on the question 'how should this trial change our opinion about this effect?' This compels the analyst to:

1 state a reasonable (defensible) opinion on the effect of A (the new treatment), excluding evidence from the trial (the 'prior distribution');
2 state the support for different values of the effect of A, based solely on the data from the trial (the 'likelihood');
3 combine these two sources to produce a final opinion about the effect of A (the 'posterior distribution').

The 'posterior' distribution is produced using Bayes' theorem which states that the posterior distribution is proportional to the product of the 'prior' multiplied by the 'likelihood'. For those wanting more detail, Spiegelhalter et al. (2000) provide an accessible overview of principles and applications of Bayesian methods to health technology assessment. They define the Bayesian approach thus: 'the explicit quantitative use of external evidence in the design, monitoring, analysis, interpretation and reporting of a study' (Spiegelhalter et al. 2000). From this definition, it can be seen that the approach can also be applied to meta-analysis and other forms of quantitative synthesis (see below).

The rationale for Bayesian methods in health and health care derives from an awareness of the limitations of traditional trial methods (e.g. the complications for trial design generated by a desire to report multiple sub-group analyses and the attendant risk of type I error (wrongly rejecting a true null hypothesis)), together with the fact that evidence from multiple sources usually needs to be combined to inform a policy decision. For example, in undertaking trials, Bayesians would allow inferences from qualitative studies about how users react to different types of therapy to inform the 'prior' distribution of outcomes as well as using such information to make recommendations about the use of a treatment trialled at a population level on specific types of individuals. The Bayesian approach thus has the attraction of allowing – potentially at least – the use of any form of relevant evidence in addition to formal randomised controlled trials. This might include, for example, qualitative data, clinical consensus statements, expert views, and stakeholder opinion as inputs to meta-analysis, quantitative modelling, and simulations of effectiveness and cost-effectiveness of interventions or policies.

Proponents argue that, as a result, a Bayesian approach is more likely to provide conclusions from syntheses of research and other information in a suitable form for making specific clinical or policy decisions in particular contexts (Dixon-Woods et al. 2001). It is likely to be particularly useful when data from primary research are weak or lacking and decisions nonetheless need to be taken in an informed and reasonable way.

Bayesian analysts explicitly bring subjective judgement into the conduct and interpretation of scientific research and evidence-based decision-making, on the grounds that ultimately decisions depend on such judgements. They then attempt to identify what it is reasonable for an observer to believe in light of the available data. By putting the subjective element into the open, it is argued that it is more likely to be amenable to rational discussion and control. This also means that a Bayesian analysis explicitly takes account of the perspective of the potential user of the analysis (e.g. whether these are pharmaceutical companies, regulators, payers, physicians, patient representatives, etc.) and draws attention to the fact that the implications of scientific research for making decisions depend on the perspective(s) adopted. Such an approach has much in common with widely accepted views among qualitative researchers that different pictures of reality will be produced by collecting data from different groups and using different methods.

What are the implications of Bayesian approaches?

The use of Bayesian decision modelling has major implications for the way in which policy-makers and managers relate to those undertaking syntheses for policy and management purposes. Firstly, it is argued by proponents of this approach to modelling that it makes little sense for policy-makers to commission the creation of a comprehensive decision analytic model unless they are prepared to use it as a direct guide to their eventual decisions. If such a model incorporates all available information, and includes values and preferences that are broadly regarded as reasonable (particularly by the decision-makers), then, the proponents argue, the output should reflect the best course of action in the circumstances from the perspective of those taking the decision. Accordingly, it makes no sense to use the output from the modelling as yet another input to a traditional implicit 'taking into account and bearing in mind' (Dowie 2006) decision. This is a radical shift in decision-making processes that many policy-makers are reluctant to embark upon. An alternative argument might be that even if those commissioning a Bayesian approach to decision modelling reject the result it may still help them to make their final decision by making the consequences of particular value positions explicit in terms of decisions they lead to. It is even possible that decision-makers may change their values when they can see the consequences.

The second major implication of attempting to bring together all relevant scientific and other information in a decision analytic model is that policy-makers have to define and explain up-front the key value judgements and trade-offs that they are prepared to make. For example, the relative weight to be given to different outcomes (e.g. reducing child poverty versus encouraging people into paid work in a welfare reform) has to be determined so it can be built into the decision analytic model. Population preferences may well be in conflict or even incoherent, in which case judgements will have to be made by policy-makers that the modellers can work with. The main practical limitation of the Bayesian approach relates to the feasibility of converting complex, implicit judgements into specific weights and probabilities, though there are methods available, for example, to convert qualitative probabilistic judgements such as 'x is extremely possible' or 'x is slightly possible' into numerical weightings (Light and Pillemer 1984: 121). It is also questionable whether decision-makers can know in advance exactly what information will become relevant to a particular decision in a specific context in order to inform the modellers and decision analysts sufficiently for them to develop comprehensive models.

Third, and related to the above point, policy-makers have to make available to the analysts (who may be in-house staff or external) all the existing information that is relevant, as well as funding the collection of extra data such as population preferences, if time and resources permit. In systems where the policy process has traditionally been confidential, the requirement for sharing information with the analysts represents a major change in relationships and ways of working.

The fourth implication relates to the analysts. In the Bayesian approach there is no neat cut-off between evidence of acceptable scientific quality and that which can be excluded. In addition, it is not sufficient for the analyst to conclude that the evidence is inadequate and leave it to someone else to cope with the decision-making consequences. The analyst/synthesizer has to produce a best solution in the circumstances with the information available.

Fifth, views, preferences and judgements have to be quantified whether from research or 'intelligence' collected more informally (e.g. from stakeholder management processes). Qualitative phrases such as 'giving x due weight', 'establishing the right balance between x and y', 'group A is strongly supportive of objective X', 'X is highly likely to be the reaction of group B to policy N', and so on, all carry quantitative and/or probabilistic implications which have to be drawn out explicitly for modelling to be possible. This is not an easy task.

Finally, a Bayesian would argue from the outset that the conclusions of all decision analyses depend on who is conducting them, for what purpose and on the basis of what evidence and opinion (i.e. context is vital). As a result, it is not possible, or desirable, to portray the eventual decision as the only 'true' one; rather it appears to be the best decision given all the material to hand to construct the model. For some policy-makers, this is an uncomfortable position to be in since it means explicitly presenting the decision in terms of uncertainty rather than the usual assumption of certainty. This has large implications for the conduct of politics as well as government processes.

Cross-design synthesis

Unlike the other synthesis methods in this chapter, cross-design synthesis can handle only quantitative data, but does allow for subjective judgements about the relevance and applicability of different sources of evidence to be brought to bear on the synthesis. It is a form of meta-analysis that allows the pooling of data from studies with different quantitative research designs (e.g. RCTs and non-randomised experiments) and the use of modelling to estimate a 'true' effect of a policy or programme, conditional on both the design of the study and the characteristics of the relevant population (US General Accounting Office 1992; Droitcour et al. 1993). The method is based on making explicit statistical adjustments to studies and modelling their likely biases in order to produce a 'true' overall estimate of effect. Instead of eliminating low quality studies from the synthesis, such studies are used where they can provide information that compensates for weaknesses or gaps in the high quality research available. For instance, many RCTs are of restricted applicability because they tend to be carried out on unrepresentative populations (e.g. excluding elderly people), so wider-ranging studies can be used to supplement the synthesis dataset as long as their potential biases are explicitly allowed for in the modelling of effects. Hierarchical modelling is used to allow for quantitative within-and-between-sources heterogeneity in the pooled dataset.

Although not a Bayesian approach per se, cross-design synthesis lends itself to Bayesian methods. It allows for a priori beliefs regarding qualitative differences between various sources of evidence to be included in the analysis. These subjective judgements are likely to be informed by a wide range of qualitative and non-research information, and are likely to be context-specific. As a result, the goal of cross-design synthesis is not to produce a universally applicable answer, but one that is 'true' in the circumstances.

Though cross-design synthesis has been applied to questions of effectiveness, this integrated form of analysis using different databases, RCTs, case-control and prospective comparative studies, leads naturally into both cost-effectiveness analysis and comprehensive decision modelling with the addition of evidence on 'utilities' and costs (see below).

Bayesian meta-analysis

Meta-analysis is a synthesis technique for the statistical pooling of the results of quantitative studies with the same or very similar designs (unlike cross-design synthesis) and focused on the same research question to calculate an overall estimate of the relative effectiveness of one intervention in comparison with another. In addition, it allows the reviewer to explore and explain the patterns in the results of different studies. Pooling of results from similar studies can be shown to reduce bias (e.g. in estimates of the effectiveness of a particular intervention) by increasing the statistical power of the analysis. With greater power, it is possible to detect small positive or negative effects. Meta-analysis is particularly useful when there is a large number of studies of similar design on the same question, where a narrative reviewer might struggle to reach a definite decision because of the complexity of the results tending in different directions. There is not space here to describe and assess meta-analysis in detail, but see Cooper and Hedges (1994: parts IV–VI) for further information.

Conventional meta-analysis is an extremely powerful tool for synthesizing the findings of quantitative studies, particularly RCTs of effectiveness, to produce a single estimate of effect and has been shown to be less susceptible to reviewers' biases than narrative approaches (Bushman and Wells 2001 cited in Petticrew and Roberts 2005: 202–3) but, it was not designed to accommodate mixed qualitative and quantitative evidence. However, recently, a Bayesian approach has begun to be applied fruitfully to the more familiar meta-analysis of RCTs and other quantitative comparative studies (e.g. of effectiveness), which allows both qualitative and quantitative data to be used together.

An example of an innovative Bayesian synthesis that draws on findings from qualitative and quantitative research is shown in Box 3.4. This study aimed to identify and assess the relative importance of a range of factors potentially affecting the uptake of childhood immunisations. The synthesis used the findings from qualitative studies of immunisation uptake to inform a prior distribution (a numerical ranking of factors affecting immunisation uptake from individual studies). These prior probabilities were combined with

---

Box 3.4 An example of a Bayesian meta-analysis of qualitative and quantitative research evidence (Roberts et al, 2002)

Objectives
- To identify factors potentially affecting uptake of childhood immunisation in developed countries
- To assess the probable effect of these factors on levels of uptake.

Methods

1   Generation of a prior distribution of factors from qualitative findings

A prior distribution of factors likely to affect the uptake of childhood immun-isation was derived from the subjective views of the researchers (n=5). This was revised after the researchers had read all relevant qualitative studies and extracted factors from each study, ranked them in order of importance and then revised their first opinions on the factors and their ranking. Rankings of each factor given by each researcher were combined to yield an overall probability that the factor would be important in determining uptake of immunisation.

2   Extraction of quantitative data

Data were extracted from quantitative studies according to categories (factors) generated by analysis of qualitative studies, with extra categories (factors) generated as needed if not included in the qualitative studies.

3   Statistical analysis

The prior probability of a factor being important was combined with the quantitative evidence to form a posterior probability that each factor (e.g. lay health beliefs) was important in affecting uptake of immunisation. Regression models for the odds of uptake were constructed using relevant data from the quantitative studies for each factor in turn.

Results

Qualitative and quantitative studies identified some common factors, but others were reported only in qualitative or quantitative studies. For some factors, addition of quantitative data substantially modified prior probabilities.

Features

Inclusion of qualitative and quantitative studies allowed a wider range of poten-tial factors affecting the uptake of immunisation to be identified and assigned a probability of importance.

Qualitative and quantitative studies contributed distinctively different evidence relevant to improving take-up (e.g. quantitative studies highlighted the effect of socio-economic factors and qualitative studies showed the importance of lay health beliefs).

probabilistic data extracted from quantitative studies and analysed together to identify and gauge the importance of a wider range of factors linked to uptake than either the qualitative or quantitative literatures could have provided alone. The study shows the benefits for policy and management of trying to include both qualitative and quantitative evidence since there were potentially important factors that would have been omitted had one or the other source of evidence been relied upon.

Bayesian approaches can incorporate qualitative findings to help identify relevant variables to include and their likely effects. These can generate quantified beliefs about the effect of variables to inform the prior probability distribution. The prior distribution can then be combined with the quantitative studies to produce a combined estimate of the effect based on all the available evidence; that is, the prior probabilities of a variable being important are modified in the analysis of the relevant quantitative studies to produce an overall, posterior distribution of probabilities. This application of the Bayesian approach allows the researchers' and/or other experts' prior beliefs explicitly to enter the analysis, but ensures these beliefs are tempered by the research evidence.

Qualitative studies contribute to Bayesian meta-analysis by identifying the variables of interest for the subsequent quantitative meta-analysis (i.e. the approach is perhaps more sequential than transformative of the original data), including possibly bringing to light some variables or factors not included in any of the quantitative studies. In the example in Box 3.4, it was clear that the integration of qualitative and quantitative research made the resultant review far more complete and revealing than either source alone could have offered. Though it is relatively simple to grasp, the Bayesian approach to meta-analysis has the disadvantage of being difficult to accomplish well since it is technically complex and may, as a result, be regarded as lacking transparency. Also it may be criticised by qualitative researchers for restricting the role of the qualitative evidence to informing the prior assumptions about variables and their effects.

Bayesian approaches to cost-effectiveness analysis

Increasingly, health economists argue that Bayesian methods are crucial for useful cost-effectiveness analysis (Luce and Claxton 1999) on the grounds that hypothesis testing is of limited relevance in economic evaluations since additional, non-trial evidence is needed to produce an estimate of the cost-effectiveness of a policy or intervention to inform a decision. This has become particularly apparent in decisions on the regulation of pharmaceuticals and medical devices where cost-effectiveness estimates of the potential advantages of innovations over existing technologies and drugs frequently have to be made ahead of definitive research findings, and/or when the innovation itself and its application are still being refined (see Box 3.5 for an example). For

---

Box 3.5 An example of a systematic review and economic decision modelling for the prevention and treatment of influenza A and B (Turner et al. 2003)

Objectives

- To establish the clinical and cost-effectiveness of available drugs for the treatment of influenza relative to the existing method (no treatment or antibiotics)
- To establish whether two of the available drugs are effective and cost-effective alternatives to the existing method of prevention (no intervention or vaccine)
- To make policy recommendations.

Methods

Systematic review and meta-analysis of randomised trials to look at effectiveness including additional evidence from pharmaceutical companies not available from the published literature. Separate reviews of evidence of effectiveness in population sub-groups (children, healthy adults, 'high risk', i.e. over 65 years with concomitant disease, and elderly people in residential care)

Economic decision models constructed to examine cost-effectiveness and cost-utility (marginal cost per Quality Adjusted Life Year (QALY) gained) of a range of feasible strategies for treating and preventing influenza, informed by the systematic reviews and other information (e.g. on likely timing of treatment after onset of symptoms in real world settings)

Estimates of the probability that costs per QALY lie within particular ranges for each strategy and for population sub-groups

Sensitivity analysis of results

Conclusions

Cost-effectiveness varies between intervention strategies and target population sub-groups. In all cases, the cost-effectiveness ratios for vaccination were either low or cost-saving. Cost-effectiveness ratios of antiviral drugs were relatively unfavourable except for some scenarios involving treatment of elderly people in residential care where anti-virals as an additional strategy could be cost-effective (i.e. 60% likelihood of cost per QALY gained below £30,000). There were a number of areas where further research could improve the modelling of cost-effectiveness.

Features

- Analysis focused on comparing a range of feasible potential treatment and prevention strategies

(continued overleaf)

Box 3.5 (continued)

- Not all comparisons had been directly studied before, but were relevant to policy decisions
- Analysis using UK-based or adjusted overseas information to produce UK-relevant recommendations (i.e. context-specific)
- Comparisons focused on marginal costs and benefits (i.e. assuming current policies exist)
- Range of research (RCTs and database studies) and non-research (expert opinion) data brought together, spanning many decades
- Results expressed in terms of their probabilities

---

similar reasons, a Bayesian approach is an attractive way of providing a quantitative estimate of the likely cost-effectiveness of undertaking research studies. Such 'value of information' studies need to take into account the likely impact on clinical practice of the results of trials and in order to do so, need to be able to estimate the probability of different trial results occurring.

A Bayesian approach can also be applied to conventional sensitivity analysis in which prior probability distributions are placed over the uncertain inputs to the analysis and the resulting distribution of potential cost-effectiveness ratios is generated by simulation. This enables the range of cost-effectiveness ratios to be presented together with the likelihood that each would in fact occur.

Comprehensive decision modelling

Systematic reviews of evidence can be built into the development of decision analyses, thereby enhancing the relevance and applicability of systematic reviews to decision-making (Cooper et al. 2002). For example, the Bayesian informed cost-effectiveness analysis discussed above can be developed into a full-scale decision-theoretic model (Dowie 2001). This is a formal, analytical means of incorporating a wider range of evidence beyond research studies into a synthesis as well as making explicit the value judgements necessary to identify the best course of action for decision-makers (with the aim of increasing the likelihood that decisions will be informed by evidence).

Comprehensive decision modelling incorporates all the major steps in a rational decision process (see Box 3.6) – synthesis of the available scientific evidence from all levels of the evidential hierarchy, valuation of the outcomes in terms of 'utilities' (e.g. quality-adjusted life years gained) and preference elicitation (defining and measuring the trade-offs between policy goals such as maximising health gain versus maximising access improvements among low users). The analysis uses Bayesian statistics together with stochastic cost-

Box 3.6 Stages in comprehensive decision modelling	
Synthesis of best available research evidence	Information on effects and costs of different policies/ programmes relevant to the particular context/ population collected and 'weighted' according to its probability of being 'true'
Valuation studies	Valuing outcomes (e.g. using time trade-off, standard gamble, etc.) to produce 'utilities'
Preference elicitation	Defining and measuring trade-offs between goals and outcomes by identifying population views (ideally from specially collected data from surveys and focus groups, but can use any other intelligence available)
Link research evidence to population preferences and valuations	
Assess costs and benefits of options and state probability of each occurring in the way predicted	

effectiveness analysis and is typically implemented using Monte Carlo simulations. It attempts to compare the costs and benefits of different programmes or interventions allowing for the uncertainty underlying the available evidence so that results can be presented to decision-makers as probabilities that each course of action or intervention is the most cost-effective. The modelling can incorporate the impact on outcomes and costs of a mix of policies or programmes operating at different levels in a system such as the simultaneous impact on smoking rates of changes in excise duty (macro), smoke-free workplace legislation (meso) and health promotion initiatives (micro).

The quality of the modelling rests on careful searching and processing of evidence relating to each parameter in the model, including explicit valuation of the outcomes (if there are more than one) and costing of each policy option. Each parameter is usually presented as a probability distribution to represent the inherent uncertainty underlying the evidence used.

Proponents argue that by making explicit the value judgements and trade-offs inherent in decisions, as well as the effect of variations in evidence quality and gaps in evidence, the approach is superior to traditional, non-analytical, implicit decision-making processes which risk overlooking important issues altogether without it being possible to know whether this has happened or not. Dowie (2006) has coined the phrase 'taking into account and bearing in mind' to summarise the conventional, largely implicit approach to decision-making and contrasts it with Bayesian decision analysis. He argues that comprehensive decision modelling may still be imperfect, but is likely to be superior to non-Bayesian approaches to decision-making since, paradoxically, it deals with all the uncertainties and trade-offs explicitly, transparently and quantitatively rather than implicitly, covertly and qualitatively.

What are the strengths and limitations of Bayesian approaches?

Perhaps the strongest aspect of Bayesian approaches to synthesis is that, at least in theory, they allow the synthesis of all available sources of evidence from RCTs, databases, professional consensus exercises, expert opinion, tacit knowledge, population focus groups, other qualitative research, etc. into a single quantitative model. Beliefs about the differences in validity between these different sources of evidence are explicitly included in the research synthesis. Such analyses try to make explicit and transparent all the judgements that have to be made to assess options and take decisions in specific contexts. They attempt to quantify the effects and costs of each potential option on the same basis. This should, in principle, improve comparison across options within a single decision, but also improve consistency across separate decisions (e.g. this may improve the allocative efficiency of government). Another benefit is that models can be updated at any time as new evidence and information on any part of the model become available, thus permitting decisions to be reviewed and if necessary revised after a period of time. Models also show clearly where the evidence to support decisions needs to be improved and can begin to show the value of new research.

Bayesian decision analyses admit to the inherent error and uncertainty of decisions since they relate, by definition, to unknowable future states. This approach strengthens accountability for decisions since it is possible for observers to assess whether the decision taken was reasonable given the parameters of the model, and to propose improvements which can be discussed. It militates against 'off the cuff', poorly informed decisions and allows explicit recognition of multiple perspectives, the perspective(s) from which the analysis was undertaken and how the results would alter if other perspectives were included. This resonates with the view of qualitative researchers who tend to argue that 'who you are, who you ask and where you sit' influence what you find and the conclusions you draw.

There are concerns that Bayesian approaches will include studies with 'weaker' designs in the synthesis, thereby potentially undermining the validity of the analysis. There are also concerns about feasibility: for example, that the biases and differences in rigour between studies are, in practice, tricky to handle in order to produce a synthesis of effects, or that even the best model cannot cope with the presence of multiple stakeholders with different utility functions which are hard to tease out and to reconcile. The risk is that the model gives an impression that we know more than we really do. The models could produce a perception that the subtleties of policy advice and decision-making are being reduced to mechanistic formulae even if this is not necessarily the case. They can be accused of undermining the role of ordinary policy-makers by putting decisions in the hands of unaccountable 'experts' in modelling. This could be seen as undemocratic, particularly if the results conflict with politicians' 'priors'. Relatedly, the complexity or specialist nature of the processes for developing the model and the models themselves can be difficult to communicate to lay audiences. Models require a considerable amount of work to assemble (e.g. to convert qualitative information into utilities and probabilities) and there may not be time or analytical capacity to do this. Finally, decision analytic approaches to using research synthesis for policy and management decision-making may indicate the need for such extensive, even revolutionary change in the way that public policy is made that they could be regarded as impractical.

The advocate's response to most or all of the above criticisms and concerns is that they implicitly compare decision analytic approaches to a perfect approach to policy and management decision-making that does not exist. For the advocate of Bayesian approaches, the argument can only be resolved through using decision analytic models and assessing the consequences of the decisions they indicate versus more traditional methods.

Qualitative comparative analysis

What is it?

The final method discussed in this Chapter was termed by its author (Ragin 1987) 'the qualitative comparative method'. However, this is a slightly misleading title for an approach that sits somewhere between qualitative and quantitative approaches to synthesis. In this method, data from case studies are summarised and compared using a set of simple algorithms based on Boolean logic, the aim being to identify the necessary and sufficient conditions across cases required to produce a particular outcome. The approach is thus a method for analysing the complex causal pathways described in different case studies of the same phenomenon in as economical a way as possible.

Ragin's experience as a comparative political sociologist trained in quantitative, multivariate methods had been frustrating. He observed that comparative social science tends to be qualitative, case-oriented and sensitive to the complexity and historical specificity of each setting, thereby making cross-case generalisation difficult. By contrast, quantitative comparative studies were hampered by the small number of observations (e.g. country case studies) available, the paucity of comparable variables and a lack of historical and cultural comparability between countries (or regions). As a result, it was impossible to test statistically the relatively complex patterns of causality shown in individual case studies. For example, it was difficult to answer questions such as: 'In which circumstances do military regimes of government collapse, given that individual case studies show that any of a number of conditions may be sufficient to prompt a collapse?' He argued that even with the more sophisticated techniques of multivariate analysis, quantitative analysis tended to assess a particular causal variable's average influence across a range of settings, but could not identify the different contexts in which a particular factor influenced a specific outcome or not (i.e. the ability to cope with complex statistical interactions was limited).

Qualitative comparative analysis was developed as a direct response to this limitation in conventional analysis and is thus a possible method for synthesizing findings across studies. It attempts to synthesize all cases of a phenomenon (e.g. military regime collapse) into a dataset so that all cases with the same outcome (e.g. regime collapse) can be explained by a parsimonious causal model using Boolean logic. The method uses what is called a 'truth table' to lay out all logically possible combinations of the presence or absence of independent (explanatory) variables related to a particular outcome variable. Data are coded into binary format (0 or 1) according to whether the variable is present or not. The literature is searched to find actual cases that match as many as possible of the combinations of independent and dependent variables. Where case studies vary in only one explanatory variable, yet produce the same outcome, this variable is considered logically irrelevant and is therefore removed. This process of Boolean minimisation reduces the number of potential explanations for the dataset.

Table 3.1 (overleaf) is a hypothetical example of a 'truth table' showing the three causes of military regime failure distributed across 22 case studies of different countries taken from the research literature. Each row represents case studies with identical combinations of the key causal variables and in each case should be viewed holistically (i.e. as a distinctive combination of variables). Thus the third row of case studies should not be interpreted as cases where 'B caused F', but cases in which 'B caused F in the absence of A and C'.

The table shows that any of the three conditions of regime collapse may be sufficient to provoke collapse and that the presence of more than one does not necessarily increase the likelihood of collapse. After logical reduction using Boolean algebra, this very simple example shows that $F = A + B + C$ since, in Boolean algebra if $A + B = Z$ and $A = 1$ and $B = 1$, then $Z = 1$; and $1 + 1 = 1$ (addition in Boolean algebra is the equivalent of the logical operator 'OR'). That is, if any of the additive terms is present then the outcome occurs (is true). For example, if someone can kill themselves in three different ways, it does not matter how many of these ways they choose to use, they will still kill themselves. So, if they put their head in a gas oven and take an overdose, they will not be 'more dead' than if they had only used one of the methods (oven or

Table 3.1 Hypothetical truth table showing three causes of regime failure (Ragin 1987)

Conditions (explanatory variables)			Regime failure (dependent variable)	No. of instances in the literature (22 case studies)
A	B	C	F	
0	0	0	0	9
1	0	0	1	2
0	1	0	1	3
0	0	1	1	1
1	1	0	1	2
1	0	1	1	1
0	1	1	1	1
1	1	1	1	3

A = conflict between older and younger military officers
B = death of a powerful dictator
C = CIA dissatisfaction with the regime

pills). Satisfy any one of the conditions and the expected outcome (death) is the same in Boolean addition.

So the Boolean equation $F = A + B + C$ represents the synthesis of the 22 case studies of the causes of military regime failure in Table 3.1 and states that failure can occur because of any one of: conflict between older and younger military officers (A); death of a powerful dictator (B); and CIA dissatisfaction with the regime (C). It appears to be no more likely to occur if more than one cause is present than if only one is present.

Table 3.2 shows another hypothetical truth table, this time reviewing 38 studies of successful strikes already in progress. The unreduced (primitive) Boolean equation for this is: $S = AbC + aBC + ABc + ABC$. To explain the notation, it is conventional in Boolean algebra to use capitals for the presence of a variable and lower case for its absence. Following Boolean minimisation of the primitive form: ABC combines with AbC to produce AC; ABC combines with ABc to produce AB; and ABc combines with aBc to produce Bc. Thus $S = AC + AB + Bc$. In other words, successful strikes occur either when A and C are present, or when A and B, or when B is present in the absence of C. This can be simplified still further to: $S = AC + Bc$, since AC and Bc cover all four of the 'primitive' expressions (ABC, AbC, ABc and aBc). Successful strikes occur either when there are both booming product markets and the strikers have a large strike fund, or when there is a threat of sympathy strikes but the strikers do not have a large strike fund.

Table 3.2 Hypothetical truth table showing three causes of successful strikes (Ragin 1987)

Conditions (explanatory variables)			Successful strike (dependent variable)	Frequency (number of
A	B	C	S	studies)
1	0	1	1	6
0	1	0	1	5
1	1	0	1	2
1	1	1	1	3
1	0	0	0	9
0	0	1	0	6
0	1	1	0	3
0	0	0	0	4

A = booming product market
B = threat of sympathy strikes
C = large strike fund

What are the strengths and limitations of qualitative comparative analysis?

This approach has many advantages. First, it is very direct compared with a statistical analysis. In a statistical analysis, a linear, additive combination of the three presence/absence variables in the first illustrative truth table would predict that cases with more than one of the three conditions would somehow experience more of a regime failure – but a regime either fails or survives. Second, to use statistical methods more cases would have been needed in association with a log-linear or discriminant analysis. The analysis would, in turn, have produced complex models because of the interactions between the variables. Third, compared to qualitative comparative case study methods, the approach allows the synthesis of a relatively large number of cases into a very economical form. Fourth, the approach is also good for identifying complex patterns of causation (what Ragin calls 'complex causal conjunctures') yet expressing them in a simple way. It starts with the most complex case studies taken in their entirety and logically simplifies their causal combinations through contrasts to produce the most parsimonious set of all 'necessary and sufficient' causes. The final advantage of the approach is that competing explanations drawn from theory and previous research can be tested. The main downside is the fact that the method seems to have been so little used so there are few examples to use as models and guides.

Summary

This chapter has discussed some of the approaches to synthesis which deal with numerical forms of data. Some of the methods described have to date only been used for 'stand alone' synthesis of quantitative evidence, others are beginning to be used to synthesize diverse kinds of evidence: all of them have the potential to do this. The key difference between the methods described appears to be the mode of analysis employed. Content analysis, case survey and the various Bayesian approaches seek to statistically interrogate or manipulate the data – whether this is in the form of frequencies (counts) or meta-analysis of some kind. Of these methods, the Bayesian approaches have particular affinity to the decision support function described in Chapter 1. The perhaps misnamed 'qualitative comparative analysis' method developed by Ragin also relies on having data in numerical form, but it is rooted in Boolean logic rather than statistical analysis. This method appears to offer considerable potential for synthesis for policy- and decision-making but there are few examples of its application in this arena.

Having looked at a number of quantitative approaches, the next chapter presents some of the main approaches which utilise qualitative (text-based) and interpretive approaches to the challenges of combining diverse sources of evidence.

4 Interpretive approaches to evidence synthesis

Chapter 3 looked at quantitative methods for synthesis. This chapter explores a group of methods which deal with qualitative (text-based) data and which have a broadly interpretive approach to synthesis. There is some overlap between the methods described in this chapter and the next in that some of the methods described in Chapter 5 in that they too use qualitative, textual evidence and do not count or statistically manipulate these data. The distinctive feature of the methods described in this chapter is that they deal with data in qualitative form and adopt an interpretive analytical approach. This approach is linked closely to the interpretive paradigm in social science, associated with the work of the the social theorist Max Weber, and the idea of *verstehen* (understanding). Interpretive social science centres on an empathetic understanding of meaning and is directed towards generating new conceptual understandings and theoretical explanations.

Understanding qualitative research methods

Before outlining the main approaches to interpretive synthesis that could, potentially, be used with a mix of qualitative and quantitative studies, it is worth briefly discussing what is meant by 'qualitative' research. Qualitative research encompasses a range of methods that can be used within different research designs. It may be stand alone or used as part of a mixed-method approach (O'Cathain and Thomas 2006) alongside quantitative methods. In addition some research strategies such as ethnography draw on more than one qualitative method. In much qualitative research the choice of research method is informed by a theoretical perspective (e.g. phenomenology, hermeneutics, ethnomethodology, grounded theory) which provides a framework for the research. The different theoretical perspectives draw on different disciplines and approaches to research, such as anthropology, sociology, social policy, political science, psychology, history and economics. The methods used to collect data in qualitative research include direct observation, interviews, the analysis of documents and the analysis of audio- or video-recorded speech or behaviour. The analytical approaches of different disciplines vary, but the common focus of qualitative research is on language and interaction, and on understanding (interpreting) meaning (Pope and Mays 2006).

Many, but not all, qualitative research studies are small scale, principally because they are not concerned with statistical generalisability, but are instead concerned with conceptual and theoretical development (i.e. explanation of phenomena). Many qualitative studies focus on a single or a small number of cases (a single setting such as a hospital, school or neighbourhood, or a work group such as a paediatric care team, or a group of patients with a particular illness.) One of the strengths of this focus in qualitative research is that it can provide analytical depth and contextualised detail. The difficulty this poses for any attempt at synthesis is whether it is appropriate to combine the results of several unique, contextually rich studies, thereby reducing the attention to depth and detail. Against this, attempts at syntheses, and wider reviewing activities, indicate that there is a lack of cumulative knowledge from qualitative research – partly because of problems in identifying qualitative studies (Dixon-Woods et al. 2001; Dixon-Woods et al. 2006a), but also because of a failure to cross-reference and cite other related studies in accounts of primary qualitative research (Pound et al. 2005). Synthesis can help to address this gap in knowledge and thereby provide support for policy- and decision-making.

Combining qualitative and quantitative evidence in interpretive synthesis

Some of the methods discussed in this chapter have been developed for the stand-alone synthesis of qualitative research findings (e.g. meta-ethnography), others have been used to synthesize qualitative and quantitative results together (e.g. cross-case analysis). We are arguing, of course, that all of these methods have the potential to be used in the synthesis of diverse evidence including both qualitative and quantitative data. One of the more common, less demanding ways of handling qualitative and quantitative findings in the same review is to conduct a synthesis of qualitative evidence in parallel with a separate quantitative synthesis. Another strategy is to use a synthesis of qualitative research findings to help answer one of the review questions that the quantitative synthesis either cannot answer or has answered only partially. Some of the synthesis methods used for these types of review are discussed in Chapter 5. If however the synthesis seeks to integrate qualitative and quantitative evidence in a single review, a way must be found to overcome the problem of converting any quantitative data into qualitative (text) form for the synthesis. That is, while it may be possible to 'quantitise' certain kinds of qualitative data for analysis (as demonstrated in the previous chapter), it is much more difficult to imagine how one would 'qualitise' quantitative data in order to turn it into the sort of rich description that could be used in one of the approaches described in this chapter. This may explain why there are fewer attempts to fully integrate qualitative and quantitative evidence in this way.

The synthesis of qualitative research and especially the synthesis of qualitative with quantitative evidence are relatively recent endeavours. As a result, most of the methods used for this type of synthesis are at a developmental stage, and, not surprisingly, there are few examples of their application. In particular there are few examples of the application of interpretive synthesis methods to the synthesis of qualitative with quantitative research findings. This is because many of the methods involved were developed to synthesize qualitative research findings alone, and not to combine qualitative and quantitative research findings. The methods available, perhaps unsurprisingly, draw heavily on the methods and analytical techniques used in primary qualitative research.

Is it feasible to synthesize qualitative evidence?

It is worth highlighting here that the synthesis of findings from multiple qualitative studies or with quantitative evidence is not only taxing to do, it is also intellectually contested. Some researchers view the synthesis of qualitative research as illegitimate on the basis of epistemological concerns (i.e. relating to theories about knowledge and how it is acquired) and ontological concerns (i.e. beliefs about the nature of reality). Systematic reviews, and by extension, synthesis, are sometimes seen as being associated with positivism and the idea that the accumulation of research findings will arrive at a single 'truth'. Many of those engaged in qualitative research, and indeed some quantitative researchers, do not adopt such a straightforwardly positivist outlook. The findings of different research studies are instead seen as providing distinct, unique views of reality, and within qualitative research especially, different research methods are seen as eliciting multiple truths such that no single study or method is necessarily seen as providing definitive or superior knowledge.

Qualitative researchers also place greater emphasis on the importance of context and the relationship between the researcher and the researched. Sandelowski et al. argue, 'The major problem yet to be resolved is developing usable and communicable systematic approaches to conducting meta-synthesis projects that maintain the integrity of the individual studies' (Sandelowski et al. 1997: 365). Those who disagree with synthesis suggest that the attempt to amalgamate the findings of individual studies ignores vital differences in the theoretical and methodological foundations of qualitative research as well as stripping out the contextual richness of individual studies (Estabrooks et al. 1994). However, while it is worth being cognisant of these concerns, these need to be balanced against the potential benefits of building a cumulative knowledge base using interpretive synthesis.

Interpretive synthesis terminology

There are many different terms used to describe the different methods and approaches to the interpretive synthesis of qualitative evidence. These terms are not always used consistently within the literature and new terms are often applied to what appear to be only subtle adaptations of existing methods. Negotiating a pathway through this terminology and the resulting confusion is not easy. The term interpretive synthesis is used in this book to denote methods which share qualitative methodology and have a particular focus on interpretation. In health policy fields, the overarching term 'qualitative meta-analysis' is beginning to gain resonance undoubtedly because of the high visibility and status of quantitative meta-analysis in health services and health policy research and has been used to describe some of the methods outlined in this chapter (see for example Feder et al. 2006). Other terms such as 'meta-study' and 'meta-synthesis' have also been used to denote interpretive approaches to the synthesis of qualitative research.

At their core, interpretive methods for synthesis entail a process of qualitative re-interpretation and re-analysis of text-based forms of evidence. One important feature of these approaches to synthesis is that they often aim for a new interpretation or theory. Thus, for example, McCormick et al. define what they call 'qualitative meta-analysis' as 'combining the results of several studies to create interpretations at a higher level of abstraction' (McCormick et al. 2003: 943) and Schreiber et al. define their 'meta-synthesis' as 'bringing together and breaking down of findings, examining them, discovering the essential features, and in some way, combining them into a transformed whole' (Schreiber et al. 1997: 314).

Whatever the terminology used, the task of interpretive synthesis is to bring together, juxtapose, re-analyse and combine the findings from several studies into a whole that ideally provides some theoretical or conceptual development that moves beyond the findings of any individual study included in the synthesis. It is possible to reduce the very many different labels used to describe methods for such synthesis into two basic types. Firstly, there are methods based on comparison informed by so called 'grounded theory' and, secondly, there are methods, notably 'meta-ethnography' that, although still employing a comparative mode, have at their core the process of translation. The latter attempts to transform interpretations offered by individual studies in such a way that they can be expressed in each other's terms, thereby enabling direct comparison of seemingly distinctive pieces of evidence.

There are a number of techniques for data handling and presentation (e.g. use of matrix displays) which can be used to facilitate the process of making comparisons between and/or translating across studies. These can potentially be used with many different methods of interpretive synthesis including grounded theory and meta-ethnography and these are outlined in the latter part of this chapter. First, however, we look at the use of grounded theory to synthesize qualitative research and describe in detail an example of a qualitative synthesis which uses the constant comparison and theoretical elements of grounded theory. The chapter then goes on to look in detail at meta-ethnography, a translation-based method, which also makes use of constant comparison.

Comparative approaches

Grounded theory

What is it?

Many of the methods for qualitative synthesis utilise, albeit not always explicitly, the analytical methods found in Glaser and Strauss's (1967) exposition of grounded theory. Since their initial collaboration, grounded theory has developed into two slightly different methods, one informed by the methodological work of Strauss, and later Strauss and Corbin (1990), and the other by separate work carried out by Glaser (see www.groundedtheory.com). Grounded theory has been much adapted, debated and misused over the past 40 years. However the two central elements of the grounded theory approach of interest here are constant comparison as an analytical method and the use of theoretical sampling to develop and test theory. Another important feature of Glaser and Strauss's formulation of grounded theory is that it is viewed as primarily inductive, such that theoretical insights are derived from, or in grounded theory terms, emerge from, the data (1967: 48).

The constant comparative method as described by Glaser and Strauss (1967: 105–11) entails comparing 'incidents' and the properties of categories identified in the data to develop theoretical generalisations. This process begins with coding or indexing each 'incident' (these might be specific terms used by participants or concepts used by the researcher) in the data into as many categories of analysis as possible. While this coding is occurring the analyst also looks through the rest of the data to compare the current incident with previous incidents, in the same and different categories and from there to compare and contrast the properties of the different categories. This 'constant comparison' enables the reduction of categories via amalgamation and delimitation which facilitates the generation of theories or explanations.

Theoretical sampling is a process whereby data collection is informed by ongoing analysis of the data, such that hypotheses or explanations are used to determine the next phase of data collection. Thus for example if the initial data suggest that there is a relationship between some phenomenon and socio-economic class or race, then the data collection would pursue sampling of individuals from diverse class or racial backgrounds to see if this idea holds true.

Kearney used grounded theory to synthesize qualitative reports of women's experience of domestic violence (2001). She searched the English language literature on domestic violence using electronic database searches and hand-searching, and found 13 studies published between 1984 and 1999. Although Kearney did not intend to focus on a single geographical area, all the studies she identified were North American. A prerequisite for inclusion in this synthesis was that the studies had a grounded theory 'orientation' rather than being specifically labelled by the authors as such. So while the individual studies were described in the published reports as using thematic analysis, phenomenology, ethnography, grounded theory or feminist methods, they all used constant comparative techniques for the analysis of their data and demonstrated the building of concepts or theory from the data.

Kearney treated each of the 13 reports as if they were individual primary data sources. She began by noting details about each study (rather as one might extract the demographic details about each interviewee in primary research) and then extracted concepts and the interpretations/conclusions offered by the authors of each study. She summarised these details in a grid to allow comparison across the cases. From here, Kearney used the three key types of coding delineated by Glaser and Strauss: substantive; axial; and selective coding. Substantive coding is the first level of coding, sometimes also called open coding and in primary research this takes the data line by line and codes each incident. In this synthesis Kearney used this type of coding to identify the concepts in each of the studies and to group these into new categories (e.g. grouping the women's statements about how domestic abuse psychologically damaged their children or threatened their own health). Axial coding attempts to flesh out the relationships between categories and Kearney used this coding to look within and across the studies to understand the nature of the categories in the individual studies and the relationships between them (e.g. identifying moments of rationalisation or realisation in the women's accounts). Selective coding focuses down onto the core category of interest and entails searching all the data, selectively sampling any new data with the specific category in mind (i.e. sampling theoretically). Kearney used selective coding to make connections or links between her categories and a core category (e.g. developing the idea of phases and components of abusive relationships and linking these to the idea of 'enduring love'). This provided the basis of Kearney's emergent theory about women's responses to domestic violence which she was then able to test by returning to the original studies to undertake further theoretical sampling, searching for confirmatory and disconfirmatory evidence.

From this analysis Kearney developed an explanation for women's responses to domestic violence based around the idea of 'enduring love'. This she argues is a process by which women are reconciled to the violence they experience in relationships. She divided this process into four temporal phases: early endurance of what appeared to be aberrant incidents of violence ('This is what I wanted'); experience of regular abuse engendering strategies such as rationalisation, denial and monitoring ('The more I do the worse I am'); then the redefinition and moves to self-preservation ('I had enough'); and finally the establishment of a new life outside an abusive relationship ('I was finding me'). The resulting synthesis provided insights for health professionals about the strategies women experiencing domestic violence adopt.

Comparative case study

What is it?

Comparative case study is a method developed by Agranoff and Radin (1991) in the field of public administration. In essence it combines Yin's (1984) multiple case study approach with elements of grounded theory, and although used, to date, for primary research only, it has potential application for the synthesis of qualitative studies if the individual studies are treated as the 'cases'. Agranoff and Radin analyse the research questions from each of their primary research cases using a grounded theory approach – comparing and contrasting the cases to develop theory (Agranoff and Radin 1991: 216). This comparative work was facilitated by standardising the data and descriptions of each case to ensure that the same data were available for each case. In the primary research they describe the researchers met as a team to share experiences (after the fieldwork in each site) and to compare the cases 'looking for commonalities across a number of cases and determining the degree of idiosyncrasy of each site' (1991: 219).

Yin (1984) describes a similar use of grounded theory in his early accounts of how to build explanations from multiple case studies. He suggests that this entails making a theoretical proposition about policy or behaviour and comparing a specific case to this proposition, revising the statement, then comparing it with another case and so on, to iteratively refine and build an explanation. He suggests that Moore's *Social Origins of Dictatorship and Democracy* (1966) is an example of this approach. This used multiple historical case studies of the transition from agrarian to industrial societies in six countries to build a general explanation of the role of different classes in these transformations. While this now classic historical text predated Glaser and Strauss's work on grounded theory, Moore's theoretical insights were derived from a synthesis of evidence using a comparative method.

Strengths and limitations of grounded theory approaches to synthesis
Grounded theory provides an approach which has considerable potential when applied to the synthesis of qualitative studies alone as the Kearney example, above, demonstrates. The linkage between grounded theory and multiple case study methods as in the comparative case study approach developed by Agranoff and Radin (1991) suggests that the approach can be fruitfully used to synthesize a number of predominantly qualitative studies (cases) and possibly extended to enable synthesis of qualitative and quantitative evidence. Like meta-ethnography, discussed below, this approach is reliant on a thorough knowledge of the principles and application of grounded theory in primary research and for this reason is perhaps unsuited to the novice in this area. It is not at all clear how one might incorporate quantitative research findings into a grounded theory approach.

Translation-based approaches

Meta-ethnography

What is it?
Meta-ethnography is concerned with conceptual translation. Translation entails the re-interpretation and transformation of the analytical and theoretical concepts provided by individual studies into one another. Meta-ethnography is an interpretive rather than 'aggregative' (Hammersley 2006, see Chapter 1, p. 16) synthesis method: it seeks to do more than simply review a set of studies and instead aims at a novel synthesis which develops new theory to explain the research findings from a set of studies. It has been used as a method for synthesizing qualitative research alone, principally in the fields of education and health care. Meta-ethnography has also been incorporated in the synthesis of qualitative research using the 'meta-study' approach (Paterson et al. 2001) and it has been modified in one study to develop a method called 'critical interpretive synthesis' (Dixon-Woods et al. 2006b) to synthesize qualitative with quantitative research findings Meta-ethnography was developed by Noblit and Hare (1988), two social scientists working on applied research in education and health care. They developed meta-ethnography in response to an education policy research-related problem. Following the civil rights movement of the 1960s, US educational policy changed to allow black and white children to attend the same schools, and between 1975 and 1979 the US National Institute of Education supported six ethnographic case studies of the impact of urban school desegregation. The findings of these studies were rich and detailed, they revealed complex issues surrounding desegregation, but it was difficult to see how the individual studies could be summarised to inform educational policy. Two attempts to produce a synthesis and policy recommendations had failed (Noblit and Hare 1988: 19–20), but

Noblit and Hare were able to use their new method to reconcile the seemingly unique and divergent accounts provided by the case studies to produce a more general theory about the circumstances in which desegregation was successful. They did this by drawing on the methods they used in primary ethnographic research.

Noblit and Hare recognised that the traditional narrative review lacked 'some way to make sense of what the collection of studies is saying' (1988: 14–15). They were also aware of the growth of 'knowledge synthesis' and the development of statistical meta-analysis for analysing the findings of randomised controlled trial data. While they were clear that such meta-analyses were identified with the positivist tradition and its emphasis on aggregation rather than interpretation, they were nonetheless interested in seeing if it was possible to combine knowledge within a qualitative tradition to similar effect. A key influence on Noblit and Hare at this time was the work of the philosopher/sociologist Stephen Turner and his theory of sociological explanation as translation. While their method was rooted in comparison of the case studies, Noblit and Hare's approach to synthesis also entailed the more ambitious translation of studies into one another. This translation is idiomatic; it focuses on the translation of salient categories of meaning, rather than the literal translation of words or phrases.

Noblit and Hare chose the term meta-ethnography to differentiate this new approach from methods for synthesizing quantitative research (e.g. meta-analysis). The term 'meta' was prefixed to indicate that this approach, whilst not seeking to generalise statistically from a group of studies, involved combining a number of studies thereby creating something different from any one of them (hence 'meta' meaning 'across'). The key difference is that they used the prefix 'meta' to refer to 'translation' rather than pooling of data. They used the term ethnography because the studies they were working with in the initial desegregation synthesis were ethnographic. There is a growing recognition that the term 'meta-ethnography' is not ideal as a general label. It has led to a false assumption that only ethnographic studies can be synthesized using this approach when in fact it is possible to use this method to synthesize the findings from a range of different qualitative theoretical and methodological approaches, as subsequent meta-ethnographies have shown.

Stages of meta-ethnography

Noblit and Hare break the process of meta-ethnography down into seven steps or stages, but it is worth noting that they are clear that these steps are iterative, so that each of the stages can repeat and overlap during the synthesis.

1 *Getting started*
   This step entails identifying the area of interest, which Noblit and Hare

suggest should be something that is 'worthy of the synthesis effort' (1988: 27).

2 *Searching and selection of relevant studies*
The next step is mapping the studies to be included. As in primary qualitative research, this searching and selection is purposive, and it may not need to be exhaustive or comprehensive since the goal is theoretical not statistical generalisation. There are likely to be some difficulties in searching electronically for qualitative studies as these may not be adequately key-worded and some of the relevant material may be in monograph form so it is worth deciding at the outset how such material will be dealt with.

3 *Reading the studies*
Repeated reading of the studies, in much the same way as one would repeatedly read raw data in a primary study is required to identify the concepts and interpretations offered by the individual studies. In effect these concepts and interpretations become the raw data for the synthesis.

4 *Determining how the studies are related*
This stage explores the relationships between the individual studies. This typically involves compiling a list of the ideas, key concepts and explanatory schema, and (initially) speculating about how these are connected to each other. As the synthesis process develops it becomes clearer how the studies are related to each other and Noblit and Hare suggest that there are three possible ways of relating and synthesizing the studies: namely when the studies are directly comparable (they term this reciprocal translation); or oppositional (refutational); or they sustain a 'line of argument'.

- Reciprocal translation entails the iterative translation of the concepts in each study into the concepts of the other studies in the synthesis. Typically there are some overarching concepts or themes which apply across each of the studies. Noblit and Hare use an example of a group of four studies about schools. While each study was about a different type of school (junior or secondary level) and different contexts (urban and suburban), it was possible to synthesize the findings to describe two types of school which operated with either a bureaucratic or a negotiated order (1988: 45–6). These key differences could then be used to explain the different stratification and status patterns of white and black students, and the different ways in which conflict was managed in the schools.
- Refutational synthesis is derived from the Kuhnian idea that

scientific knowledge progresses through argument and counter-argument. Refutational synthesis therefore can encompass a study designed to refute an earlier study, or studies which adopt competing disciplinary or ideological perspectives. While Noblit and Hare map out this form of synthesis with two examples, one drawn from the field of education, the other a controversy in anthropology, there are few examples of this form of synthesis in the literature.

- Line of argument synthesis is based on inference. This examines what we can say about the whole based on the individual studies included in the synthesis. Again this resembles primary qualitative research, in as much as it is about building theory from the individual studies. The key difference in synthesis is that an extra hermeneutic or explanatory level is added (i.e. a new interpretation and understanding). In primary research the researcher provides an interpretation of the data, but in a synthesis the person conducting the synthesis provides another interpretation of the previous set of interpretations. The development of lines of argument shares processual elements with theory building in the grounded theory approach as well as having similarities with clinical inference, as Noblit and Hare acknowledge. Lines of argument are developed from the translated studies by comparing and sorting interpretations, examining similarities and differences, and then integrating or framing these within a new interpretation that can be applied across all the studies. As Noblit and Hare explain, the aim of a line of argument synthesis is to 'discover a "whole" among a set of parts' (1988: 63).

5   *Translating the studies into one another*
The fifth stage compares the studies by looking at similarities and differences between the concepts. This is where the translation element occurs, in as much as the person conducting the synthesis asks if one concept can be mapped onto another and scrutinises any conceptual differences. The logical sequence of the translation becomes 'A is like B except . . .'

6   *Synthesizing the translations*
This takes the translated concepts from step 5 to identify concepts which transcend individual accounts and which can be used to produce new interpretation or conceptual development.

7   *Expressing the synthesis*
The final step is to find ways to communicate the synthesis (see Chapter 6 for a fuller discussion of some more aspects of presentation).

While Noblit and Hare concede that most syntheses are expressed in written form they note that other forms (video, artistic) may have potential for such expression, depending on the purpose of the synthesis and the audience. Given the centrality of translation to the meta-ethnographic endeavour it is no surprise that Noblit and Hare emphasise the importance of ensuring that the product of a synthesis using this method should be intelligible:

> The focus on translations is for the purpose of enabling an audience to stretch and see the phenomena in terms of others' interpretations and perspectives. To do this means we must understand the audience's culture in much the same way as we understand the studies to be synthesized; we must represent one to the other in both their commonality and their uniqueness.

Noblit and Hare emphasise that undertaking meta-ethnography requires previous experience in qualitative methods. The inductive nature of the process means it is emergent, in that the initial question or area of interest may be adapted or redirected and there are numerous judgements to be made along the way which the novice is likely to find difficult if not impossible to make. They also note the influence of the person conducting the synthesis in the process, acknowledging that his or her values and readings of the studies will influence the synthesis, and inevitably provide just one possible interpretation of what are already interpretations of interpretations.

To date, meta-ethnography has primarily been used for qualitative synthesis, in education (e.g. Rice 2002; Doyle 2003), health (e.g. Jensen and Allen 1994; Paterson et al. 1998; Campbell et al. 2003; Clemmens 2003; Walter et al. 2004; Pound et al. 2005; Smith et al. 2005), and to examine literatures on topics such as leadership (Pielstick 1998) and e-government (Siau and Long 2005). Two linked meta-ethnographies of medicine-taking behaviour provide illustrations of the use of this method to synthesize published qualitative research.

Meta-ethnographies of medicine-taking

Britten et al. (2002) provide a demonstration of the meta-ethnographic approach synthesizing four qualitative studies relevant to the question 'How do the perceived meanings of medicines affect patients' medicine-taking behaviours and communication with health professionals?' They identified the common and recurring concepts in each paper (preserving the interpretations offered in the original papers) and displayed these in a matrix to enable systematic comparison and translation of the studies into one another. This led to the development of new interpretations which they referred to as 'third order interpretations'. This borrowed Schutz's (1962) ideas about different levels or 'orders' in the construction of meaning to suggest that if the primary data are 'first order' (i.e. the research participants' interpretations), then the researchers' interpretations are 'second order' and those doing the synthesis provide a third order interpretation (see Box 4.1). Britten et al. translate the concepts across the four papers to construct a line of argument that there were two quite distinct forms of medicine taking, one adherent to instructions and one based on self-regulation.

These ideas were developed further in a second, larger synthesis reported by Pound et al. (2005) which used meta-ethnography for a synthesis of medicine-taking based on 37 papers whose primary focus was patients' views of medicines prescribed and taken for the treatment of a long- or short-term condition (excluding medicines taken only for preventive purposes). Pound et al. (2005) searched the literature over a ten-year period 1992–2001, using a combination of electronic and hand-searching methods. They describe how they found it necessary to add two further steps to Noblit and Hare's process for meta-ethnography. As a way of organising the reading and translation of the studies they organised the papers into seven medicine groups and initially translated the studies into each other within these groupings. They explored how the studies were related within groups before moving on to determine how the studies were related across groups. Finally they synthesized the translations across all the medicine groups (see Box 4.2).

The process of reciprocal translation entailed determining how the concepts proposed in one study could be expressed in relation to those used in another study. For example, a paper by Britten (1996) had conceptualised unorthodox accounts as those accounts provided by patients that were critical of medication (i.e. they viewed it as unnatural and damaging); critical of doctors; and generally active rather than passive. It was possible to map or translate this concept onto the ideas about self-help and moral repertoires

---

Box 4.1   Example of second and third order interpretations (Britten et al. 2002 adapted)

Second order interpretations	**Third order interpretations**
Patient undertakes own cost benefit analysis of treatment. Medicine-taking influenced by cultural meanings & resources	Self regulation includes the use of alternative coping strategies
Self regulation limited by fear of coercion	Self regulation flourishes if sanctions are not severe
Patients may not express views which they do not perceive be medically legitimated	Alternative coping strategies are not seen by patients as medically legitimate. Fear of sanctions and guilt produces selective disclosure

---

Box 4.2   Phases in the meta-ethnography of medicine-taking (Pound et al. 2005)

1   Topic selection
2   Searching for the studies
3   Reading and appraising
4   Organising studies into medicine groups
5   Translating studies within medicine groups
6   Determining how studies are related within groups
7   Determining how studies are related across groups
8   Synthesizing translations across medicine groups
9   Reconceptualising findings

---

offered by Lumme-Sandt et al. (2000) which differentiated accounts according to which people said they preferred natural remedies, had strong negative views about medication and did not obey doctors versus those in which people stressed that they took only a little medication, used it responsibly and moderately, and when explaining why they needed medication, gave reasons beyond their control.

By systematically repeating this reciprocal translation process Pound et al. (2005) developed a series of 'illness maps' which depicted how the various concepts in the studies were related (see example in Figure 4.1). These were then synthesized to develop a model of medicine-taking which encompassed all the studies included in the synthesis (see Figure 4.2). They proposed a line

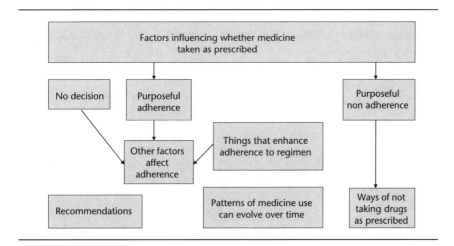

Figure 4.1   An example of an illness map from the medicine-taking meta-ethnography (Campbell et al. forthcoming)

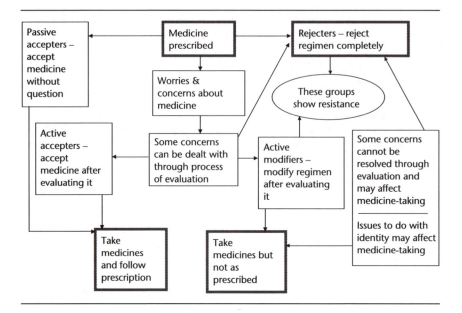

Figure 4.2 Model of medicine-taking (Pound et al. 2005)

of argument that medicine-taking (or rather failure to take medicines) could be understood by using the concept of 'resistance' as a way of explaining patients' responses to prescribed medicines. This captured both the passive and active responses by patients and the wide range of strategies employed in relation to taking medicines (or not) reported in the original studies.

Critical interpretive synthesis – a variant of meta-ethnography

To date there has been only one study which has attempted to synthesize qualitative and quantitative research using a variant of meta-ethnography. This method has been called 'critical interpretive synthesis' (Dixon-Woods et al. 2005; 2006b). As well as extracting the key concepts or interpretations from a large number of qualitative studies this method 'extracted' similar concepts and themes from quantitative papers, principally from the discussion and conclusion sections of such papers and grey literature. The extracted concepts were compared across all the studies using a thematic analysis and constant comparison. The researchers supported this analysis with some of the charting and matrix type techniques outlined at the end of the chapter and with qualitative analysis software. Box 4.3 describes the approach in more detail.

Box 4.3   An example of critical interpretive synthesis (Dixon-Woods et al. 2006b)

Dixon-Woods et al. (2006b) conducted a large synthesis of a diverse literature on access to health care by vulnerable groups. This was based on 119 qualitative and quantitative papers sampled from over 1200 potentially relevant studies. The synthesis was based on meta-ethnography but the authors found that working with such a large and diverse set of papers meant that they had to re-specify and adapt meta-ethnography to the extent that they decided to give the resulting method a different name.

Working in a large multidisciplinary team, the authors developed a data extraction chart which was used to record the concepts and key findings from each paper along with a summary description of the study and methods. The researchers identified key themes and compared these across the studies included in the synthesis. From this, they were able to identify recurring themes and categories that helped to explain access to health care. They also sought to provide a critique of the literature being synthesized, for example, questioning the assumptions and categories used in the original papers. The product of this synthesis was a 'line of argument' about access to health care which described how access was jointly negotiated and accomplished between health services and their users. This centred on the concept of *candidacy* which 'describes how people's eligibility for health care is determined between themselves and health services. Candidacy is a continually negotiated property of individuals, subject to multiple influences arising both from people and their social contexts and from macro-level influences on allocation of resources and configuration of services'.

Strengths and limitations of meta-ethnography

Meta-ethnography suffers from the same general problem facing all systematic reviews of qualitative evidence that the qualitative literature is not well recorded or indexed on the main electronic bibliographic databases. There are also issues to be resolved relating to inclusion and quality appraisal of qualitative studies (see Chapter 2). The closeness of meta-ethnography to methods used in primary qualitative research means that it requires a high level of expertise in qualitative methods since 'translation' requires interpretation and judgement. One way of examining the validity of the interpretations offered by meta-ethnography is to send the results of the synthesis back to the researchers involved in the original studies (much like respondent validation in primary qualitative research (Bloor 1997). Doyle (2003) reports doing this successfully in a synthesis, but this practice may be as problematic as it has proved in primary research. For example, in primary research if respondents dispute the interpretation offered by the researcher this does not automatically invalidate the researcher's perspective since the researcher and the participants in a study occupy different social roles, have different experiences of the same phenomena and are likely to interpret events differently. Similarly the interpretation offered by those undertaking synthesis is unlikely directly to match the views of the original researchers since the reviewers' theory is based on the whole range of studies available. Meta-ethnography has, to date, only been used to synthesize research evidence but it may have potential to include more diverse forms of evidence, especially text-based evidence.

Techniques for comparing studies in an interpretive synthesis

Grounded theory and meta-ethnographic methods for synthesis both require careful comparisons to be made between the studies included in the synthesis to identify concepts and themes which are common or similar across the studies. This section of the chapter looks at how matrices or charts can be helpful in facilitating such comparisons. Miles and Huberman (1994: 172) describe a range of approaches to qualitative data analysis within primary research which they call 'cross-case analysis' or 'synthesis' which can be employed to facilitate these kinds of comparisons. Several of these entail the matrix or chart display as a way of dealing with multiple cases and these techniques can be fruitfully applied to the synthesis of multiple studies.

Miles and Huberman (1994) use what they describe as a 'meta-matrix' which entails first examining each whole case (study) in detail, then developing case-based matrices to display specific variables from individual cases, then displaying the cases together in a meta-matrix to allow systematic comparisons. Faced with an unwieldy dataset, the analyst can standardise and reduce the data by sorting, quantifying and collapsing them into analytic categories which can be displayed together on larger meta-matrices (in essence, theme x case charts). Matrices can be created with varying levels of complexity, for example, ordering material by cases, or by themes (variables), or displaying the data chronologically, or looking at two variables together and pulling out multiple exemplars for comparison and so on. Miles and Huberman detail some 27 different ways of constructing matrices each of which provides different viewpoints on the data, but some possible templates are illustrated below (Figure 4.3).

Two examples of synthesizes which have used matrix-based techniques are McNaughton (2000) and Lloyd Jones (2005), both in the context of nursing research. McNaughton used Miles and Huberman's approach to conduct a synthesis of 14 qualitative studies looking at public health nurses making home visits to mothers of young children. She used this to identify common elements across the studies to develop theories about nurse visiting. Lloyd Jones (2005) used matrices in a synthesis of 14 qualitative studies about role development for nurses. Of these, Lloyd Jones' approach is perhaps the more interesting as it utilised the 'framework' approach for primary qualitative

Simple case x theme matrix

	Theme A
Case 1	
Case 2	
Case n	

Chronological tabulation of cases

	Time 1	Time 2	Time 3
Case 1			

Cross tabulation of variables or themes

	Variable/theme 3	Variable/theme 4
Variable/theme1		
Variable/theme 2		

Figure 4.3 Examples of matrix displays (Miles and Huberman 1994 adapted)

analysis (Ritchie and Lewis 2003). The framework approach has five stages (which share features of both the comparative and translational approaches to interpretive synthesis described above):

1 familiarisation with the data and/or studies (i.e. reading and re-reading)
2 identification of a thematic framework, typically derived form the research questions
3 indexing or coding of the data/ and/or studies
4 charting (i.e. transfer of summaries to matrix displays)
5 mapping and interpretation.

Lloyd Jones (2005) used framework analysis to extract and summarise information about barriers and facilitators to various specialist and advanced nursing roles and these were displayed in a thematic matrix which shows how the barriers and facilitators are shaped by such things as the characteristics of the postholder and the organisation, and the relationships between those in the 'new' role and other members of the team (see Table 4.1). She went on to

Table 4.1 Example of a thematic matrix-based comparison as part of synthesis (Lloyd Jones 2005)

Theme	Facilitators	Barriers
Characteristics of the postholder	Confidence Ability to accept responsibility Ability to make decisions Optimism Conflict resolution skills Adaptability Flexibility Stamina Assertiveness Negotiating skills Change management skills Proactive facilitative expert practitioner style Political astuteness Motivation Creativity (to develop the role) Forward-looking Good interpersonal skills Consistency in values and behaviour Individual characteristics match job	Lack of confidence Emotional over-involvement with patients
Postholder's previous experience	Substantial previous experience in the specialty Clinical expertise Previous employment in the same hospital Prior knowledge of the specific service	Lack of networks in the hospital Lack of experience in the specialty
Professional/educational issues	National professional/educational issues • Clear career pathways and professional development	National professional/educational issues • Perceived ambivalence of professional regulatory bodies in relation to the role • Absence of educational standardization for role

Table 4.1 *(continued)*

Theme	Facilitators	Barriers
		• Lack of clear career pathways and professional development
		• Grading and pay too low relative to responsibilities
		• Lack of medico-legal clarity
	More local issues	More local issues
	• Formal higher education	• Lack of relevant courses
	• Knowledge base in the relevant specialty	• Lack of induction to the role
	• Clinical preparation for role	• Lack of role models and mentors
	• Generic preparation for role (including research skills, time management skills, etc.)	• Loss of generalist skills
	• Flexible educational pathway	• Lack of appropriate appraisal and supervision
	• Reading about the role and its development	
	• Keeping up-to-date	
	• Maintaining clinical competence	
	• Induction to the role	
	• Training posts	
	• Role models	
	• Appropriate appraisal and supervision	
	• Feedback	
	• Reflective practice	
	• Performance measurement	
Managerial/organiza-tional issues	Culture of employing institution	Culture of employing institution
	• Institution values clinical expertise	• Organizational culture and agenda
	• Size of hospital/specialty	• Organization slow to change
		• Short-term contracts, lack of forward planning

(continued overleaf)

Table 4.1 *(continued)*

Theme	Facilitators	Barriers
	Role definitions and boundaries • Clear role definitions and boundaries • Autonomy • Protocols (useful only to the less experienced)	• Size of hospital/specialty Role definitions and boundaries • Lack of clear role definitions and boundaries • Unclear expectations of role • Incompatible expectations of role • Unrealistic expectations of role • Work overload • Increasing workloads • Increase in administrative tasks • Lack of autonomy
Relationships with others	Effective interprofessional relationships Collaborative relationships with key stakeholders Support (general) Support from other specialist and advanced Support from colleagues Support from medical staff Support from nursing staff Support from managers (including nurse managers) Support from other hospital staff Support from formal counsellor Support from professional organization Support from family and church	Lack of effective interprofessional relationships Lack of support (general) Lack of support from medical staff Lack of support from managers (including nurse managers) Opposition from medical staff Opposition from GPs Opposition from managers Medical staff resistant to change Resistance or opposition from nursing staff Isolation

Table 4.1   *(continued)*

Theme	Facilitators	Barriers
Resources		Lack of resources (general)
		Lack of suitable accommodation
		Nursing staff shortages
		Lack of administrative support (including secretarial support and computers)
		Lack of full-time funding for role
		Lack of resources for research
		Lack of resources for education

argue that poor team relationships and role ambiguity were key, interrelated factors limiting the implementation of new specialist nursing roles.

Although Miles and Huberman describe using matrix techniques for qualitative data alone, and this is how McNaughton and Lloyd Jones have used them, it is possible to use matrices or charts to display and compare information derived from quantitative studies, or other sources of evidence. In their variant of meta-ethnography, termed critical interpretive synthesis, Dixon-Woods et al. (2006b) used electronic charts in a common software package to manage and display themes and concepts summarised from the commentary and discussion sections of quantitative reports.

Summary

This chapter has outlined methods for interpretive synthesis. All of the methods described have a strong comparative component, but the meta-ethnographic approach augments this with a process of 'translation' across studies to synthesize the findings of research. Given the centrality of comparison to grounded theory and meta-ethnographic approaches, the chapter also outlined some matrix-based techniques for facilitating comparisons between studies.

In primary research, interpretive approaches are principally associated with qualitative studies and it is unsurprising therefore that most of the existing examples of interpretive synthesis have focused on qualitative research alone. Of these methods, meta-ethnography probably has the strong-est record of application to the synthesis of qualitative research evidence. The lack of interpretive syntheses which combine qualitative and quantitative evidence may also reflect the difficulty of transforming quantitative evidence into qualitative form, noted earlier in this chapter. Although this is not theoretically impossible, the mixed methods approaches to synthesis con-sidered in the next chapter have sought to more directly tackle the problem of synthesizing qualitative and quantitative evidence.

5   Mixed approaches to evidence synthesis

This chapter describes some approaches to evidence review and synthesis that do not readily 'fit' into the categories described in the previous two chapters. The approaches described here are all capable of accommodating a diversity of types of evidence: quantitative and qualitative; research and non research, etc. They are, however, more eclectic than the approaches already described – an eclecticism that is evident in practice in a number of ways. For example, thematic analysis is the most common analytical method in these approaches, but a wide range of other techniques and presentational devices may be employed. More importantly, they differ markedly in the extent to which the processes for review and synthesis are systematic and transparent. The nature of the synthesis product also varies widely. In some cases, such as much narrative synthesis, the approach stops short of the formal integration or re-interpretation of different evidence sources, aiming rather to juxtapose findings from multiple sources and highlight key messages from a body of literature. In other cases, such as realist synthesis, however, the approach may involve a 'higher order' synthesis resulting in the production of new knowledge and/or theory through a process of integration and/or re-interpretation of the original studies (much the same as in meta-ethnography in Chapter 4).

This chapter is divided into four main sections. The first covers thematic analysis which is commonly used in a wide range of reviews of complex bodies of evidence. In the middle two sections, two broad but different approaches to evidence synthesis are described: realistic synthesis and narrative synthesis. The former is strongly interpretive aiming to develop new theory to explain a body of evidence. The latter is less interpretive in ambition and allows for the use of a range of different techniques (e.g. including thematic analysis) unified by the fact that the synthesis is text-based. In the final section of the chapter, a very obviously 'hybrid' approach to evidence review developed by the EPPI Centre at the Institute of Education in London is presented in which parallel systematic reviews are conducted addressing different but related elements of an overall review question. These separate reviews include different types of evidence and adopt different methods for synthesis. The results of these separate reviews are then brought together in a final 'meta-synthesis'.

Thematic analysis

What is it?

Thematic analysis is one of the most common methods for synthesis adopted in many approaches to evidence review. It comprises the identification of the main, recurrent or most important (based on the specific question being answered or the theoretical position of the reviewer) issues or themes arising in a body of evidence. It is typically the method used for identifying, grouping and summarising findings from included studies in 'first generation' literature reviews (see Chapter 1) and is commonly used in the early stages of a narrative synthesis (see below, this chapter). Though thematic analysis is primarily qualitative in origin, themes can be counted and tabulated (much as in 'content analysis' described in Chapter 3). However, it is perhaps more common for a thematic analysis than a content analysis to be developed, at least partially, in an inductive manner; that is without a complete set of a priori themes to guide data extraction and analysis from the outset.

Thematic analysis tends to work with, and reflect directly, the main ideas and conclusions across a body of evidence, looking for what is prominent rather than developing 'higher order', new explanations for findings that do not appear in any of the published accounts of individual studies (this contrasts with approaches such as meta-ethnography described in the previous chapter or realist synthesis, discussed below).

Themes are identified by reading and re-reading the included studies using what is essentially the comparative process described in Chapter 4. Themes can be simply coded at first, for example, by annotating the original papers, and then extracted either using 'select and copy' functions in common software programmes if the files are stored electronically, or summarised by the reviewer. The types of matrix-based techniques described at the end of Chapter 4 can be helpful ways of presenting thematic analysis.

While thematic analysis is typically associated with qualitative or text-based material, it is potentially possible to include quantitative data. This could be achieved by 'qualitising' the data, for example, in the way that Dixon-Woods et al. (2006b) extracted themes and findings from quantitative evidence for an interpretive synthesis (see Chapter 4); it is possible, having identified themes, as suggested above, to count the frequency with which they occur.

The emerging list or set of themes can be refined by identifying key themes and sub-categories. The level of sophistication achieved by this method can vary; ranging from simple descriptions of all the themes identified – often a format for 'first generation' literature reviews – through to analyses of how the different themes relate to one another (as for example in Lloyd Jones' (2005) identification of barriers and facilitators to specialist nursing roles discussed in Chapter 4).

What are the strengths and limitations of thematic analysis?

The advantage of thematic analysis is that it provides a means of organising and summarising the findings from a large, diverse body of research. It can also handle qualitative and quantitative findings since it is, in large part, a narrative approach. This means it can be used in almost all circumstances. However, as with unsystematic literature reviews, the flexibility of thematic analysis is associated with a lack of transparency. It can be difficult for the reader to be sure how and at what stage themes were identified. For example, it can be hard to judge whether the review would have looked different if an entirely deductive, theoretically-driven approach had been used instead of an inductive approach in which themes 'emerge' from the process of analysis. This uncertainty reflects the fact that thematic analysis can be undertaken in different ways (i.e. quantitatively or qualitatively; inductively or deductively; theoretically driven or descriptively). It is also unclear whether the findings from thematic analysis should reflect the frequency with which each theme is reported or its explanatory significance (content analysis suffers similarly – see Chapter 3).

Realist synthesis

What is it?

Realist synthesis is a broad approach to evidence review that focuses primarily on 'testing' the causal mechanisms or 'theories of change' that underlie a particular type of intervention or programme. Realist synthesis is therefore concerned exclusively with the question of 'what works', but it adopts a very different approach to answering this question than the Cochrane-style systematic effectiveness review (see Chapter 1). A realist review aims to test the explanatory power of the underlying theories of change shared by different interventions or programmes, asking whether and why these interventions/ programmes work (or not) for particular groups in particular contexts. Pawson (2002; Pawson and Bellaby 2006) developed this approach as an alternative to what he argued to be the two main modes of evidence review – the traditional, 'first generation' literature review and the Cochrane-style systematic effectiveness review – which he suggested had serious deficiencies that limited their value to policy and practice. He argues that realistic synthesis represents a 'third' model with particular advantages for decision-makers.

Realist synthesis can include a diverse body of evidence, including, but not restricted to, research on the causal mechanisms underlying interventions and/or programmes, and the contexts in which these are implemented in order to answer the question: 'What works, for whom, in what circumstances?' The rationale for realistic synthesis is theory-building according to the scientific principle of 'falsification' (Popper 1959). According to Popper, the mark of good science is a commitment to testing the limits of its explanations: when analysis reveals an exception or limit to a theory, the existing explanatory framework must be revised to accommodate the exception. In principle, realist synthesis involves the systematic review of a series of different programmes or interventions all resting on the same underlying causal mechanism designed to tease out precisely how these seemingly distinct programmes work and why they work differently in different contexts.

Pawson and Bellaby (2006: 88) describe the process of realist synthesis as follows:

> The researcher begins with program A, which is discovered to work in certain ways for certain people. The 'findings' are accepted because the reviewer can produce a theory of how it works. This explanation is then applied to program B. If B performs as predicted, then an expansion of the scope of the theory is demonstrated. However, if there are mixed results (a more likely outcome), there must be an amendment and re-specification of the theory. In theory this process can continue indefinitely but time and other resources are likely to determine the number of comparisons that could be undertaken.

An example of realist synthesis in miniature

Pawson and Bellaby (2006) have produced what they refer to as a 'miniature' realist synthesis of evidence on the effectiveness of peer support programmes. Peer support has been used as a mechanism to address a wide variety of social and psychological problems such as depression, unemployment, drug misuse, AIDS/HIV awareness, chronic illness, alcoholism, child abuse, teenage pregnancy and so on. As this example makes clear, the point of comparison in realist synthesis is the programme mechanism or theory of change: in all these programmes the underlying mechanism through which change is believed to happen is that peers will offer participants mutual support on the basis of sharing ideas and experiences, and this will ameliorate the harmful effects of difficult events, change problem behaviour and generally improve psycho-social functioning.

Like other approaches to evidence synthesis, the realist approach extracts data from various sources of evidence (which in this instance can include research or non-research sources such as newspapers or official reports). The purpose of data extraction is to identify the explanations offered for change across different policy domains and any underlying patterns of success and failure that reoccur. The ultimate aim of the review is to use these data to develop a theory about the conditions (or contextual factors) that 'determine' the success or otherwise of the particular programme mechanism – in this case, peer support.

Steps in a realist synthesis of peer support (summarised from Pawson and Bellaby 2006)

1 *Fathers* Recent burgeoning interest in fathers and fatherhood has produced a number of father-focused demonstration projects and programmes, like the Texas Fragile Families Initiative and Parents Fair Share programme, aimed at supporting young men toward becoming good providers, caretakers, and ultimately committed fathers for their young families. Support groups have been a popular mechanism toward achieving this goal.

   A review of research reveals that the outcomes of these efforts have been mixed. Whilst charismatic professional leadership can result in sustained active participation on the part of fathers, it has been difficult to find these leaders and when turnover of leaders is frequent or the quality of leadership is poor, peer group membership drops. Attendance is also a problem as young men's lives can be somewhat chaotic and complex with many demands on their time. Although young men report that they enjoy the interaction and increasing their knowledge through participation, they find regular attendance difficult.

   In a realist synthesis, a reviewer would identify useful information about the need for charismatic leadership (contextual factor one or C1) and the constraints of complex networks and schedules (C2) so establishing the first steps of a theory of peer support group efficacy.

2 *Unemployment* Unemployment is associated with social isolation, depression and anxiety or, at very least, stress. Job clubs are argued to provide emotional support and opportunities to network with others, helping participants learn pre-employment 'etiquette' and problem solving skills.

   Research suggests that the outcomes for this application of peer support have also been mixed. Job clubs that are flexible offering varied times for meetings which mesh well with erratic schedules are better attended. These clubs are matching peer-group programmes to peer-group lifestyle – this provides the reviewer with positive evidence to reinforce the initial contextual theory.

Research also shows that club participants who receive training to increase their skills, in addition to peer support, are more likely to find a new job with better pay than those receiving support alone. The realist reviewer could use these data to develop the hypothesis that peer support may be limited in its application to chronic or structural problems (C3).

Research suggests that a participant who has not completed high school will not find a well paid job as a result of peer support group participation. So the reviewer may extend the developing theory to suggest that in the face of such chronic problems as low educational attainment, peer support appears to be effective only as a part of, or as a conduit to, a more comprehensive programme including concrete interventions (C4).

3 *Chronic illness* Peer support is also common as a part of a treatment plan for people with chronic illnesses. It is argued to provide not only the reassurance to participants that they are not alone in coping with their condition, but may also serve to improve physical health and mental well being.

As with job clubs, research suggests that peer support for people with chronic illness appears to be more effective in conjunction with other interventions such as individual psychotherapy and family psycho-education – thus adding weight to contextual hypotheses (C3 and C4).

However, in contrast to the other programmes, research suggests that people with chronic illnesses will go to great lengths to meet their peer mentors, regardless of difficult schedules and mobility restrictions. Given this evidence, the realist reviewer would need to modify the developing theory about adapting programmes to sub-jects' schedules (C1). The reviewer would begin to construct explan-ations for this exception. For example, it may be that peer support programmes compete with other interests or needs amongst young fathers and unemployed people, but for people with chronic illness, peer support may present a rare opportunity to make social connec-tions or may be highly valued because chronic illness is the most important issue in their lives at the time. This explanation might lead to another development of the theory (C5) to the effect that urgency and strength of need for support is another influential condition.

In the example, Pawson and Bellaby go on to look at other contextual conditions that appear to mediate the success of peer support programmes for people with chronic illness and also in relation to sexual health programmes. They eventually produce the list of contextual conditions in Box 5.1.

Box 5.1   Contextual constraints on peer support (Pawson and Bellaby 2006)

- Need for charismatic leadership (C_1)
- Fit with networks and schedules of subjects (C_2)
- Avoidance of larger, deep-seated or structural problems (C_3)
- Inclusion of a more comprehensive program package (C_4).
- Identifying and addressing urgency of support requirements (C_5)
- Identifying and addressing shared needs across the group (C_6).
- Identifying and addressing shared motivations across groups (C_7)
- Taking account of the legitimacy of peer group influence (C_8)

This outline realist synthesis serves to illustrate the process involved in developing a theory about the appropriate use of peer support groups based on an appraisal of the successes and failures of a number of diverse programmes. This theory consists of a series of contextual conditions that seem significant for the success of these programmes (summarised in Box 5.1), albeit that these conditions are not independent or additive. For example, most peer support programmes seem to require subsidiary professional interventions. But what these might be and the extent of the need for them depends on having a close understanding of the existing levels of competence of individuals within the membership of the group. It is, however, clear from this review that peer group programmes share common mechanisms for change, and the factors enabling and/or constraining their success also repeat themselves in different policy domains.

Strengths and weaknesses of realist synthesis

Realist synthesis can accommodate an enormous diversity of evidence including qualitative and quantitative research findings, material from newspapers and unpublished reports, routine statistics, etc. It can also produce compelling 'stories' that may have a unique authenticity for policy-makers and practitioners speaking to their own personal and professional experience. However, although an attractive idea, there are very few worked examples of this approach and all of the examples in the literature have involved the developer. In defence of the approach, it is possible to see realist synthesis providing a way of adding rigour and structure to the traditional, 'first generation' literature review while retaining the ability of the best of these to present arguments about the mechanisms of programme success or failure and about the apparently conflicting results of similar studies. However, the generalisability of the approach remains to be tested.

Narrative synthesis

What is it?

The term 'narrative synthesis' is used here to refer to an approach to evidence synthesis that relies primarily on the use of words and text to summarise and explain the findings of multiple studies. Whilst narrative synthesis can involve the manipulation of statistical data, the defining characteristic is that it adopts a textual approach to the process of synthesis. It has been suggested (Dixon-Woods et al. 2004: 12) that different types of evidence synthesis can be located along a continuum from quantitative approaches, which involve the pooling of findings from multiple studies (e.g. meta-analysis), to qualitative approaches, which involve an interpretative approach (e.g. meta-ethnography). Narrative synthesis lies between these two. It will always involve the 'simple' juxtaposition of findings from the studies that have been included in the review. However, where the evidence allows, it can also involve some element of integration and/or interpretation.

Variants of narrative synthesis are widely used in work on evidence synthesis, including Cochrane reviews. Even when specialist methods, such as meta-analysis, is used to synthesize findings from multiple studies, a narrative synthesis approach will often be used in the initial stages of a review. Recognising this, the guidance on undertaking systematic reviews produced by the NHS Centre for Reviews and Dissemination at York University suggests that reviewers should first undertake a narrative synthesis of the results of the included studies to help them decide which other methods are appropriate (NHS Centre for Reviews and Dissemination 2001).

However, unlike some other approaches to evidence synthesis, narrative synthesis does not rest on an authoritative body of knowledge or on reliable and rigorous techniques developed and tested over many years. In the absence of such a body of knowledge there is, as the Cochrane handbook suggests (http://www.cochrane.org/resources/handbook/index.htm) 'a possibility that systematic reviews adopting a narrative approach to synthesis will be prone to bias, and may generate unsound conclusions leading to harmful decisions'.

These problems are not, of course, restricted to narrative approaches as statistical techniques have produced biased and misleading results in the past (and continue to do so from time to time). However, there is currently no consensus on the constituent elements of narrative synthesis and the conditions for establishing trustworthiness – notably a systematic and transparent approach to the synthesis process with safeguards in place to avoid bias resulting from the undue emphasis on one study relative to another – are frequently absent. Given this situation it is perhaps not surprising that narrative synthesis is sometimes viewed as a 'second best' approach for the synthesis of findings from multiple studies, only to be used when statistical meta-analysis or another specialist form of synthesis (such as meta-ethnography for qualitative studies) is not feasible.

In an attempt to improve quality, Popay and colleagues with funding from the UK Economic and Social Research Council have produced guidance on the conduct of narrative synthesis. They argue that narrative synthesis can be used in systematic reviews addressing a wide range of questions and, therefore, including very diverse sources of evidence, but the guidance focuses in particular on the conduct of narrative synthesis in reviews of evidence on the effectiveness of interventions and those concerned with evidence on the barriers and enablers to implementation of interventions.

The guidance itself was based on a systematic search and review of literature on methods for evidence review. It offers a general framework for narrative synthesis consisting of four elements: theory development; development of a preliminary synthesis; exploring relationships in the data; and testing the robustness of the synthesis product. The purposes served by each of these elements in relation to reviews of effectiveness and of evidence on programme implementation are set out in Table 5.1.

Although the elements are separated out in Table 5.2 for clarity, the authors of the guidance are at pains to point out that reviewers will move iteratively among the activities making up these elements. For elements 2–4, the guidance describes a number of tools and techniques that may be utilised during the synthesis process. These are described in more detail in Table 5.2.

The authors include practical illustrations of the application of their narrative synthesis approach to reviews of evidence on effectiveness and implementation. These examples highlight how the choice of a particular tool and/or technique will depend on the type of evidence being synthesized.

Strengths and limitations of narrative synthesis

Methods for narrative synthesis are being developed and are beginning to address many of the drawbacks of traditional narrative reviews (see Chapter 1). The approach retains the flexibility of the traditional, 'first generation' literature reviews, being appropriate for a wide range of review questions and allowing for the inclusion of wide-ranging and disparate types of evidence (i.e. research and non-research). The narrative synthesis framework provided in the ESRC guidance has the potential to produce a more transparent and more sophisticated narrative synthesis than has been the case in the past (Popay et al. 2006). It also provides a context in which to make choices about which specific method or methods for synthesis should be adopted. Additionally, many of the synthesis tools/techniques described in the guidance are relatively simple and straightforward to use although in some cases reviewers may need training particularly where specialist techniques such as reciprocal translation of studies into each other are to be used.

Table 5.1   The purpose of the main elements in a narrative synthesis (Popay et al. 2006)

Main elements of synthesis	Effectiveness reviews	Implementation reviews
1. Developing a theoretical model of how the interventions work, why and for whom	To inform decisions about: • the review question and what types of study to review • the interpretation of the review's findings • how widely applicable the findings might be	To inform decisions about: • the review question and what types of studies to review • the interpretation of the review's findings • how widely applicable the findings might be
2. Developing a preliminary synthesis	To understand the nature of the effects by defining patterns or types of effects To organise findings from included studies to describe patterns across the studies in terms of: • the direction of effects • the size of effects	To organise findings from included studies in order to: • identify and list the facilitators and barriers to implementation reported • explore the relationship between reported facilitators and barriers
3. Exploring relationships in the data	• To consider the factors that might explain any differences in direction and size of effect across the included studies	• To consider the factors that might explain any differences in the facilitators and/or barriers to successful implementation across included studies • To understand how and why interventions have an effect
4. Assessing the robustness of the synthesis product	To provide an assessment of the strength of the evidence for: • drawing conclusions about the likely size and direction of effect • generalising conclusions on effect size to different population groups and/or contexts	To provide an assessment of the strength of the evidence for drawing conclusions about: • the facilitators and/or barriers to implementation identified in the synthesis • generalising the product of the synthesis to different population groups and/or contexts

A variety of analytical methods – appropriate to the review question and the evidence to be synthesized – can be utilised within the narrative synthesis framework, as can evolving methods for the management of larger numbers of studies and for the complex process of study quality appraisal. The use of multiple and mixed tools and techniques in the synthesis has the potential to provide novel insights into the evidence being reviewed. It will always be the case that different reviewers using the same tools and techniques to synthesize the same body of evidence in a process of narrative synthesis may produce different results. However, the narrative synthesis approach does provide a formal, auditable process to address the potential biases introduced through decisions on what research to include and exclude, and/or the synthesis process itself. Hence, it should produce more reliable and generalisable conclusions than traditional literature reviews. At the very least, the process of a particular synthesis can be challenged and, if necessary, modified.

Notwithstanding these strengths, a narrative synthesis also has some important limitations. Some of the tools and techniques have the potential for misuse. For example, the use of multiple approaches to synthesize the same data may also open up the possibility for bias through so called 'data dredging'; that is, over-interpreting the data. Another important limitation of narrative synthesis is that at present it has not been extensively practised and fully worked through examples of the use of the guidance produced by Popay et al. (2006) have yet to be published in journals. However a demonstration review using narrative synthesis is forthcoming (Arai et al.)

In an important sense, narrative synthesis is a general framework within which a wide range of specific methods for synthesis can be used and how reviewers make decisions about the appropriate methods to use in their review is a question that needs further exploration. Above all else, narrative synthesis highlights the importance of judgement in the conduct of reviews of diverse evidence sources and, therefore, the need for experience and caution on the part of the reviewers. Whilst the guidance produced by Popay et al. may increase the transparency of this approach, it does not make it any easier to reach definitive 'bottom line' conclusions about the 'story' a body of evidence has to tell. Reviewers still need to be creative in the interpretative work that lies at the heart of all evidence synthesis. The key purpose of the narrative synthesis is the organisation, description, exploration, and interpretation of the study findings and the attempt to find explanations for (and moderators of) those findings.

'Horses for courses': techniques for narrative synthesis

The guidance on the conduct of narrative synthesis described above identifies a wide range of techniques from the methodological literature that can be used to synthesize the findings of multiple studies, many of which are also utilised in the synthesis methods described in earlier chapters and some are discussed in more detail in Chapter 6 which deals with the organisation and presentation of synthesis results. The appropriate choice of techniques will depend upon the nature of the evidence being synthesized. The techniques described in the narrative synthesis guidance are shown in Table 5.2, but it should be stressed that this is not a comprehensive list; and some of the tools/techniques mentioned below exemplify a wider range of slightly differing approaches. A fuller description of these tools and techniques and narrative synthesis in general can be found in Popay et al. (forthcoming).

Combining separate syntheses: the EPPI approach

The final approach to the review and synthesis of diverse sources of evidence to be described in this chapter is that developed by the Evidence for Policy and Practice Information and Co-ordinating (EPPI) Centre at the Institute of Education in London. This approach typically involves a very broad review question from which separate sub-questions are developed. These form the focus of two or more parallel systematic syntheses. These parallel syntheses may, for example, focus on sub-questions about effectiveness, appropriateness, barriers and enablers to implementation, and the perspectives of the group targeted by the intervention. The results of the separate syntheses are then combined in a so-called 'meta-synthesis' aiming to address the review question in its entirety. It is argued that because the EPPI approach aims to address review questions that include, but are not restricted to the effectiveness of a specific intervention or programme, they are more appropriate to the needs of policy-makers and managers than the conventional Cochrane-style effectiveness reviews.

Examples of the EPPI approach to evidence synthesis have involved a series of systematic reviews synthesizing evidence on the barriers to, and facilitators of, health and healthy behaviour amongst young people (Harden et al. 2001; Oliver et al. 2001). The main steps in this series of EPPI reviews are shown in Figure 5.1. As can be seen, the EPPI approach includes all of the standard stages of a systematic review: setting the review question; developing a review protocol; searching for studies across a range of bibliographic sources; applying inclusion and exclusion criteria; assessing methodological quality; extracting data; and synthesizing findings. However, there are two key innovative aspects to this approach. First, rather than a tightly structured search strategy, the EPPI approach begins with a comprehensive mapping and quality screening exercise to identify and describe all the types of studies falling within the broad remit of the overall review question. In the context of the EPPI reviews of health and healthy behaviour amongst young people, the results of this mapping were used with a stakeholder group including the funders of the work to refine the review question. For example, the mapping exercise

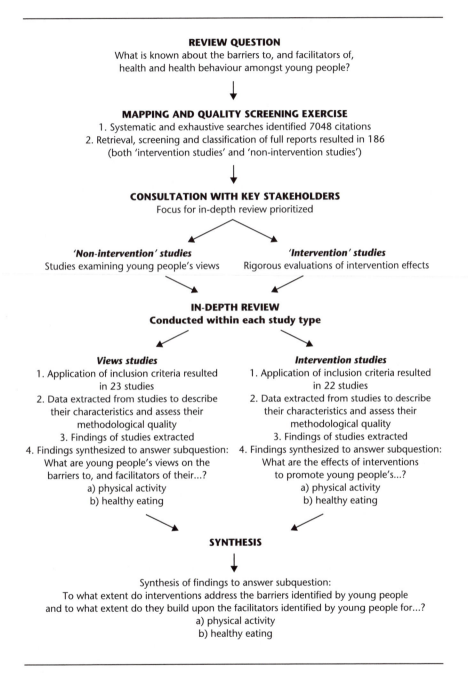

Figure 5.1 Main steps in an EPPI Centre review of mixed method evidence (Oliver et al. 2005 adapted)

Table 5.2 Tools and techniques that can be used in narrative synthesis (Popay et al. 2006 adapted)

Tool/technique	Description
I. Developing a theory: the guidance does not include any specific tools or techniques to support this aspect of a synthesis process.	
II. Developing a preliminary synthesis	
Textual descriptions of studies	A descriptive paragraph on each included study – may be useful for recording purposes to do this for all excluded studies as well. These descriptions should be produced in a systematic way, including the same information for all studies if possible and in the same order.
Groupings and clusters	Reviewers may group the included studies at an early stage of the review, though it may be necessary to refine these initial groups as the synthesis develops. Can also be a useful way of aiding the process of description and analysis, and looking for patterns within and across these groups. It is important to use the review question(s) to inform decisions about how to group the included studies.
Tabulation	A common approach, used to represent both quantitative and/or qualitative data visually (see Chapter 6). The way in which data are tabulated may affect readers' impressions of the relationships between studies, emphasising the importance of reviewers attempting some narrative interpretation of tabulated data.
Transforming data into a common rubric	When extracting data from quantitative studies, it is standard practice to extract the raw or summary data from included studies wherever possible, so a common statistic can be calculated for each study (e.g. odds ratios or standardised mean differences). In a narrative synthesis, study results will not be pooled statistically, but will allow the reviewer to describe the range of effects.
Vote-counting as a descriptive tool	Simple vote-counting might involve the tabulation of statistically significant and non-significant findings. Some reviewers have developed more complex approaches, both in terms of the categories used and by assigning different weights or scores to different categories (see Chapter 6). However, vote-counting can disregard sample size and be misleading. So, whilst this can be a useful step in a preliminary synthesis, the interpretation of the results must be approached with caution and these should be subjected to further scrutiny.

Table 5.2 *(continued)*

Tool/technique	Description
Translating data: thematic analysis	A common technique used in the analysis of qualitative data in primary research (see Chapter 4), thematic analysis can be used to identify systematically the main, recurrent and/or most important (based on the review question) themes and/or concepts across multiple studies (see above, this chapter). The process can be associated with a lack of transparency – it can be difficult to understand how and at what stage themes were identified. It is important that reviewers give as much detail as possible about how a thematic analysis was conducted.
Translating data: content analysis	Defined as 'a systematic, replicable technique for compressing many words of text into fewer content categories based on explicit rules of coding' (see Chapter 3). Unlike thematic analysis, it is essentially a quantitative method, since all the data are eventually converted into frequencies, though qualitative skills and knowledge of underlying theory may be needed to identify and characterise the categories into which findings are to be fitted.

III. Exploring relationships

Graphs, frequency distributions, and plots	There are several visual or graphical tools that can help reviewers explore relationships within and between studies, although these are typically only useful in the context of quantitative data. These include: presenting results in graphical form; plotting findings (e.g. effect size or factors impacting on implementation) against study quality; plotting confidence intervals; and/or plotting outcome measures. Frequency distributions, funnel plots, forest plots and L'Abbé plots are other possibilities (see Chapter 6 for examples).
Moderator variables and sub-group analyses	With quantitative data, analysis of variables which can be expected to moderate the main effects being examined by the review. This can be done at the study level, by examining characteristics that vary between studies (such as study quality, study design or study setting) or by analysing characteristics of the sample (such as groups of outcomes, or participants), based on some underlying theory as to the effects of those variables on outcomes.

(continued overleaf)

Table 5.2 *(continued)*

Tool/technique	Description
Idea webbing and conceptual mapping	Using visual methods to help to construct groupings and relationships (see Chapter 6). The basic idea is (i) to group findings that reviewers decide are empirically and/ or conceptually similar and (ii) to identify (again on the basis of empirical evidence and/or conceptual/ theoretical arguments) relationships between these groupings.
Translation: meta-ethnography	Translation focuses on seeking a common rubric for salient categories of meaning, rather than the literal translation of words or phrases (see Chapter 4). *Reciprocal translation* is the iterative translation of concepts in each study into the concepts of other studies. *Refutational synthesis* occurs when accounts are oppositional (in practice there are few examples of this form) and *'line of argument'* synthesis examines similarities and differences between cases to integrate them in a new interpretation that 'fits' all the studies.
Qualitative case descriptions	In general terms any process in which descriptive data from studies included in a systematic review are used to try to explain differences in statistical findings, such as why one intervention outperforms another (ostensibly similar) intervention or why some studies are statistical outliers. This kind of descriptive information may or may not be reported in the original study reports. The textual descriptions of studies described earlier would be a potential resource for this type of work.
Investigator/methodological/ conceptual triangulation	Approaches to triangulation focusing on the methodological and theoretical approaches adopted by the researchers undertaking the primary studies included in a synthesis. For example, investigator triangulation explores the extent to which heterogeneity in study results may be attributable to the diverse approaches taken by different researchers. This involves analysing the data in relation to the context in which they were produced, notably the disciplinary perspectives and expertise of the researchers producing the data.

IV. Assessing the robustness of the synthesis

Weight of Evidence (e.g. Harden and Thomas 2005)	Relevance criteria are set for a particular review and studies are then assessed for relevance using these. Those that are judged to be relevant are then assessed for methodological quality.

Table 5.2 *(continued)*

Tool/technique	Description
Best Evidence Synthesis (BES) (Slavin 1995)	Only studies meeting minimal standards of methodological adequacy and relevance to the review are included, and information is extracted in a common standard format from each study, with a systematic approach to the assessment of study quality and study relevance. This approach is not prescriptive about the study designs which can to be included in a review – this can vary, depending on the review question. It has been suggested however that BES is simply an example of good systematic review practice.
Use of validity assessment, e.g. CDC approach (Centers for Disease Control and Prevention 2005)	In this approach, the reasons for determining that the evidence is insufficient are: A. Insufficient designs or executions, B. Too few studies, C. Inconsistent, D. Effect size too small, E. Expert opinion not used. The categories are not mutually exclusive. Many other health care evidence grading systems use a similar approach.
Reflecting critically on the synthesis process	The synthesis should include a critical discussion, covering such points as: methods used (especially focusing on limitations and their influence on the results); evidence used (quality, validity, generalisability) – with emphasis on the possible sources of bias and their potential influence on results of the synthesis; assumptions made; discrepancies and uncertainties identified; expected changes in technology or evidence (e.g. identified ongoing studies); aspects that may have an influence on the implementation of the technology and its effectiveness in real settings. Such a summary would enable the analysis of robustness to temper the synthesis of evidence as well as indicating how generalisable the synthesis might be.
Checking the synthesis with authors of primary studies	Britten et al. (2002) suggest consulting the authors of included primary studies in order to 'test' the validity of the interpretations developed during the synthesis and the extent to which they are supported by the primary data. This is most likely to be useful where the number of primary studies is small. There is no reason why the primary study authors should agree with the way in which their findings have been combined with other researchers', but they may, nonetheless, have useful insights into the possible accuracy and generalisability of the synthesis.

suggested that the review would be best focusing on healthy eating and physical exercise because of the volume and quality of the evidence in these two areas compared with other areas of health and health behaviour in relation to young people. The studies identified were then grouped, according to their methodological focus, into two main study types: (i) 'intervention studies' which could potentially identify effective, ineffective and harmful interventions for promoting physical activity and healthy eating; and (ii) 'non-intervention' studies which described factors associated with physical activity and healthy eating. Two parallel reviews were then conducted: an effectiveness review; and a review of the perspectives of young people themselves on barriers to and facilitators of health in their age group.

The second innovative element of the EPPI approach is the final meta-synthesis when the results of the parallel syntheses are brought together to address the overall review question(s). This stage of the EPPI approach to synthesis involves the development of a matrix in which the findings from the parallel syntheses are juxtaposed. This process does not involve the pooling or integration of synthesis findings since they are from very different types of studies: rather the process has been described as one of building up a mosaic of findings to produce an overall picture from the different pieces of evidence.

In the series of reviews described in Figure 5.1, the final 'meta-synthesis' involved comparing the mainly qualitative findings on young people's views about the factors (barriers and enablers) that influenced their health and behaviour now or could do so in the future with the interventions and outcomes focused on in the effectiveness studies. This allowed the review team to explore two questions: (1) to what extent did interventions address the barriers to healthy eating and physical exercise identified by young people and (2) to what extent did interventions incorporate the factors that young people identified as facilitating healthy eating and physical exercise? In other words, the meta-synthesis focused on the extent to which the interventions that had been evaluated could be argued either to diminish barriers identified by young people and/or build on the facilitators. An example of part of a meta-analysis matrix is shown in Table 5.3.

On the basis of their analysis, the reviewers made the following recommendations:

- When soundly evaluated interventions were effective and matched young people's views, they were recommended for implementation.
- When other interventions matched young people's views but were unclear in their effects, they were recommended for further development and evaluation.
- When gaps were apparent, they recommended that new interventions be developed and tested.

Table 5.3 Example of a 'meta-synthesis matrix from an EPPI Centre review (Oliver et al. 2005)

Young people's views of evidence of effectiveness

barriers/facilitators	from soundly evaluated interventions	from other interventions	recommendations
The school			
Consultation of choice of physical activities	No matching evaluations identified	Increased range of activities including aerobics and dancing	Evaluate further interventions that make physical education programmes more appealing, with more choices
Lack of healthy choices in school canteen	Provision of more fruits and vegetables for school meals: 'Gimme 5' programme effective for reported healthy eating: North Karelia Youth Programme effective for healthy eating behaviour, reducing systolic blood pressure and modifying fat content of school meals: Slice of Life effective for reported behaviour, practical skills, awareness and knowledge	Two interventions changing the cooking practices of school canteen staff (e.g. using less salt and fat)	Increase the availability of healthy foods in school and complement with classroom activities and media campaigns
Practical and material resources			
Creation of more cycle lanes	No matching evaluations identified	No matching evaluations identified	
'Fast food' is cheap and easy to access: 'healthy food' is expensive and difficult to access	No matching evaluations identified	No matching evaluations identified	

The strengths and limitations of the EPPI approach

The EPPI approach to evidence review has a number of significant strengths. Perhaps the most important from the perspective of this book is that it utilises a larger proportion of research and potentially other literature relevant to a review question. It is also clear that the review questions that have been addressed using this approach are broader in focus than is often the case with evidence reviews and hence are more likely to be relevant to the complex and often wide ranging concerns of policy-makers and managers (see Chapter 8). This approach can involve any number of parallel but linked syntheses addressing different questions about, for example, subjective perceptions of need, intervention design and development, acceptability and feasibility, as well as (cost) effectiveness. It also provides a transparent path from evidence synthesis to recommendations for policy action and for future research. However, this is also a time-consuming and expensive approach to synthesis, requiring large teams of reviewers to be dedicated to the work for long periods of time. This in itself may be a constraint on its utility for policy.

Conclusion

To the extent that there is any commonality in the three broad approaches to synthesis described in this chapter (thematic analysis, realist synthesis and narrative synthesis), it is that they are less well codified than other approaches making fewer pre-specified demands on reviewers. Whilst some approaches – narrative synthesis, for instance – provide a clearly delineated framework for reviewers to operate within, typically they all leave the choice of specific methods for synthesis to the reviewers. This flexibility can be an advantage, but it also requires a great deal of care on the part of reviewers and arguably a considerable amount of experience of evidence synthesis if a good quality review is to be achieved. Both realist synthesis and the EPPI approach are also demanding of time and human resources. The challenges for reviewers that arise from the lack of clearly defined 'rules for synthesis' in these approaches – particularly realist synthesis – are compounded by the lack of well worked through examples. This is likely to change in the future, but for the moment both realist and narrative synthesis remain in an important sense 'experimental'.

PART 3
The product of evidence synthesis

This section of the book looks at the product of synthesis. It is interested not only in the use of the finished outputs of synthesis for policy- and decision-making, but also how the results of the analytical process can be summarised and presented effectively. Chapter 6 looks at organising synthesis as part of the process of doing synthesis as well as for the final product of synthesis. It discusses how to plan these aspects of synthesis and the kinds of content that might be needed in different kinds of report. It describes some of the different methods for displaying and summarising material from a synthesis and outlines some of the currently available software to support the analysis and presentation phases of synthesis and reviewing. Chapter 7 looks at the issue of using synthesis to inform policy- and decision-making. This re-examines the different reasons for using knowledge from research and other kinds of evidence in policy- and decision-making, by considering the differences between the 'enlightenment' and rational models of the use of research. This chapter also looks at how policy gets made in practice, exploring possible barriers and facilitators to the use of synthesis in this context. Chapter 8 draws together the approaches and methods for synthesis and review for policy- and decision-making discussed in the rest of the book. It discusses how to choose appropriate approaches to synthesis in different situations and suggests a way of appraising the quality of syntheses and reviews.

6 Organising and presenting evidence synthesis[1]

This chapter outlines different techniques for organising and presenting the various interim and final 'products' of a synthesis. Like the other elements of the synthesis process discussed in this book, the business of writing up is not easy. It is important to recognise that successful presentation is a skill, and is partly a creative process and partly reliant on careful planning.

A core reason for presenting synthesis (or any research) is to inform those who might or perhaps should use the findings. As noted in Chapter 1 the dissemination of the results of a synthesis can help to overcome the problems associated with relying on a single study or piece of evidence and is a way of helping policy-makers and managers make their way up the information 'mountain'. Sharing this accumulated or integrated knowledge can be useful for a range of different decision-makers in policy, management and practice, and of course it will also be useful to researchers. A second reason for organising and presenting the synthesis process and findings clearly is to ensure and demonstrate that the review has been rigorous and is of high quality. Once completed, it will be vital to give an account of the methods and process of the synthesis. Taken together, these accounts should meet the test of transparency, providing an open and honest description of how the findings were arrived at. To this end, much of the material in this chapter is about different ways of organising the interim and final findings in a synthesis to facilitate the process of synthesis and as a way of providing a transparent record of the process in retrospect.

Thinking about organising synthesis materials and how to communicate the findings of the synthesis or review should begin early in the design and planning stage. The way the results are presented should be directly linked to the research questions, the scope and the content of the synthesis, and, of

---

[1] This chapter includes a synopsis of material from Popay, J., et al. (2006) *Guidance on the Conduct of Narrative Synthesis in Systematic Reviews*; Version 3: A Product from the ESRC Methods Programme. Available from the Institute for Health Research, Lancaster University, UK.

course, the rationale for conducting the synthesis in the first place. It is important to consider how the results will be disseminated and to whom, and indeed to discuss different possible strategies for this with those who are likely to be trying to use the findings or help others take notice of them. Petticrew and Roberts note that 'knowledge sharing is a two way process, and if end point users have been involved in setting the research questions, and have participated in advisory groups, some of the work of dissemination will already have been done' (2006: 256). However, often there will be multiple audiences for a review or synthesis who cannot be communicated with face-to-face or informally. For example, it may be possible to keep in relatively close contact with the funders or commissioners of a review and even some of the managers or policy-makers who may be planning to take its conclusions into account, but there will be other officials and the wider research community who cannot be reached in this manner, in which case a way needs to be found of making sure that the results are disseminated to each relevant constituency. The style and format chosen for presenting findings may need to be carefully tailored to these audiences.

Planning presentation

Successful presentation of the findings of the synthesis relies on good preparation and organisation. This means keeping clear and accurate records all the way through the process of conducting the synthesis which will make it possible to reconstruct this process. This entails keeping meticulous accounts of such things as the search strategies employed, and the decisions made about methods and data analysis. If storing these items electronically, it is always worth having a back-up on disk or another computer/network as reconstructing 'lost' search strategies, for example, at the writing up stage, can be a time-consuming process.

In much the same way that a primary researcher may keep a field diary during the research process so it is also possible to record how the synthesis was conducted, including making notes about the rationale for decisions on the scope of the review, inclusion and exclusion of studies, any areas of disagreement during the analysis and how these were resolved and so on. Moreover, for those contemplating another synthesis this record can provide some indication of just how long different tasks can take – for example, that literature searching took six months and included a number of false starts.

It helps to organise and structure notes and records as much as possible during the review, for example, keeping the selected studies in alphabetical order in a file with their related decisions so that it is easy to refer back to them. Short standardised summaries of the different studies should be made and referred to during the writing up phase. It also helps to plot the narrative or 'story' of the synthesis in advance of the final analysis to provide some structure for the argument, even if this changes frequently in light of the stages in the analysis of the evidence.

Recording the searches

Keep a list of the keywords and terms used in searches, and record the sequence and development of the search strategy. As well as any electronic searching you may need to keep details about hand-searching and references collected from other sources such as suggestions from colleagues or experts contacted during the search. A record needs to be kept of the papers excluded from the synthesis and the reasons for these exclusions. These details can often be presented in technical appendices to reports and papers (see Box 6.1).

Box 6.1   Some examples of electronic search strategies for a review of support for overseas qualified nurses working in Australia (Konno 2006)

Review question: What supportive interventions assist overseas nurses to adjust to Australian nursing practice?

The search covered 1985–2003 and alongside these electronic searches the author searched reference lists of retrieved articles and relevant web sites (2006: 85). A total of 64 papers was identified and 52 of these were excluded.

Search terms
CINHAL
1   exp Australia/or (Australia$).mp
2   exp nurse/or (nurse$).mp
3   (overseas qualified$).mp
4   (migrant nurse$).mp
5   exp foreign nurse/or (foreign nurse$).mp
6   1 and 2 and 3
7   1 and 4
8   1 and 5
9   6 and 7 and 8

Medline
1   exp Australia/or (Australia$).mp
2   2exp nurse/or (nurse$).mp
3   exp emigration and immigration/or (immigration$).mp
4   (overseas qualified$).mp

(continued overleaf)

Box 6.1 (continued)

---

5   (migrant nurse$).mp
6   (foreign nurse$).mp
7   1 and 2 and 3
8   1 and 2 and 4
9   1 and 5
10   1 and 6

ERIC
1   Australia*
2   nurse*
3   overseas qualified*
4   immigration* or migration* or immigra* or migra*
5   Foreign nurse*
6   1 and 2 and 3
7   1 and 2 and 4
8   1 and 5
9   6 and 7 and 8

Dissertation Abstract
Australia? AND ((foreign nurse?) or (migrant nurse?) or (overseas qualified nurse?))

Summarising the data extraction and analysis processes

For the papers included in any synthesis it is important to produce charts or tables summarising key details about each study such as authors, year, design, methods, sample/setting, main results and, where necessary, results of any formal quality appraisal. During the synthesis these summaries may spread across more than one table, but a condensed version or parts of these records are often useful components, or in appendices to, written reports about the synthesis.

Alongside this it is also worth keeping a record of the scope and coverage of the synthesis; for example totalling up the number of participants or settings in the original studies as this can be used in reporting to provide some indication of the volume and range of evidence covered by the synthesis and, therefore, its potential generalisability and applicability.

Visual displays of synthesis material

As earlier chapters have suggested, there are different ways of displaying details about the studies included in the synthesis to facilitate comparison. Some of these can be useful in presenting the results of a synthesis too.

Tabulating details about the study designs

In the initial phases of a synthesis, tables can be used to display details of study design, results of study quality assessment, outcome measures and other results. These data may be presented in different columns in the same table or in different tables (e.g. one table for the basic description of each study and another for a quality appraisal of each study in relation to specific questions to be answered). Used thoughtfully, tabulation can be a valuable tool and can provide important building blocks for future elements of the synthesis process (Mulrow and Cook 1998; Burls et al. 2000; Evans 2002b).

Some authors stress the need to take care with the layout of tables, arguing that the way in which data are tabulated may affect readers' impression of the relationships between studies. For example, 'placing a results column adjacent to any of the characteristics or quality columns could invite speculation about correlation and association' (Burls et al. 2000). These notes of caution point to the importance of providing a narrative interpretation of all tabulated data (Hedges and Olkin 1985; Evans 2002b).

Table 6.1 is taken from a systematic review of research on the impact of social support interventions on long-term health outcomes. Hogan and colleagues (2002) concluded that, across a variety of types of social support and different health concerns, there was evidence that social support did improve long-term health outcomes. The example focuses on studies of individual interventions where support was provided by family or friends. In their narrative, the authors provide a paragraph on each of the studies identified, outlining what the study sought to do, summarising the findings and identifying any methodological concerns that might affect the interpretation or trustworthiness of the results. Commenting on the table, the authors state that:

> the observed effectiveness of including spouses and/or family members in treatment as a source of support is encouraging but it is unknown whether the inclusion of the natural support network in treatment actually increases perceived support or makes a unique contribution to treatment success.
>
> (Hogan and colleagues 2002: 405)

This approach to tabulation, involving some description of the studies, the brief articulation of any concerns or limitations, and a generic summary statement in the text, is a common approach to linking narrative text and tables in a synthesis involving small numbers of studies.

Vote-counting as a descriptive tool

Although some commentators have argued strongly against 'vote-counting', calculating the frequency of different types of results across included studies

Table 6.1 Individual interventions that provide support through family and/or friends (Hogan et al. 2002 excerpt)

Authors and sample	Support intervention	Design	Measure of support	Results
Dadds and McHugh (1992) – 22 single parents of children with conduct problems	Child Management Training (CMT) with adjunctive ally support. Allies were family members/friends of parents instructed to give emotional/instrumental support.	Random assignment to standard CMT or CMT with adjunctive ally support.	Perceived Support Scale Family and Friends (Procidiano & Heller, 1983)	Improvements observed in both groups at posttreatment and at 6-month follow-up. No additional gains observed in the adjunctive ally condition. Perceived social support was not greater in the ally condition than in the CMT-alone condition.
Hughes, Hymowitz, Ockene, Simon, and Vogt (1981) – 4103 male smokers	Behavioral smoking intervention from Multiple Risk Factor Intervention Trial. Spouse smokers invited to join as source of support and positive reinforcement.	Random assignment to treatment or control group. 6–8-year follow-up.	No	Smoking intervention demonstrated higher self-reports of abstinence and lower thiocyanate levels in the support group than in the control group.
Keller and Galanter (1999) – 30 cocaine-dependent patients (10 in treatment, 20 in control)	Network Therapy; 48 session, 24-week substance abuse therapy. Family/friend support, CBT-relapse prevention techniques, and community reinforcement.	Ten patients seeking treatment served as treatment group; control group consisted of other cocaine-dependent controls.	No	Network Therapy patients had significantly less positive urinalysis than standard treatment patients.

can be a useful way of producing an initial description of patterns in the included studies (Hedges and Olkin 1985; Cwikel et al. 2000). In the case of systematic reviews of effectiveness, a simple approach to vote-counting would involve the tabulation of statistically significant and non-significant findings as in Table 6.2. This example shows a very basic synthesis using a simple positive versus negative or equivocal vote count in which studies of the efficacy of drug treatment for irritable bowel syndrome are grouped according to intervention type. In this example statements are also made about the 'balance of evidence and recommendations'. The vote count is also presented separately for all available trials and for 'high quality' trials separately, thereby drawing attention to the need to consider the quality of evidence in each direction as well as its quantity.

Table 6.2 Efficacy of pharmacological interventions in treatment of irritable bowel syndrome (Jailwala et al. 2000)

Intervention	Global or symptom improvement		Global improvement		Balance of evidence and recommendations
	Total trials	Positive trials	Total trials	Positive trials	
Bulking agents:					
All trials	13	4	11	4	Efficacy not clearly established
High quality trials	7	3	7	3	
Smooth muscle relaxants:					
All trials	16	13	12	9	Beneficial for
High quality trials	7	7	5	4	abdominal pain

Some reviewers have developed more complex approaches to vote counting, tabulating the characteristics of the studies and assigning different weights or scores to them, as in Table 6.3. This is an abridged table taken from a Cochrane review of the effects of acupuncture on idiopathic headache. Here, the vote-count for each study not only makes a distinction between statistically significant effects and 'no difference', but also between statistically significant results and non-significant results that favour one group over another. The reviewers explain:

> Because it had been anticipated that a quantitative meta-analysis might not be possible, at least two independent reviewers voted in the following categories as a crude estimate of the overall outcome of each study:

Table 6.3 Acupuncture vs. other interventions: results for frequency and intensity (Melchard et al. 2004 excerpt)

Study	Ahonen 1984	Carlsson 1990	Doerr-Proske 1985	Gao 1999	Hesse 1994	Wylie 1997	Heydenreich 1989b
Diagnosis	(tension-type headache; TTH)	(TTH)	(Migraine)	(Migraine)	(Migraine)	(TTH)	(Migraine) (needle acu vs. acupuncture-like TENS vs. drug therapy)
Frequency measure	< 2 days/week with headache	5-step rating scale	mean % reduction headache days	Not measured?	number of migraine attacks (mean difference acupuncture vs. metoprolol, with 95% CI)	days with headache	mean % reduction headache days

Intensity measure	visual analog scale	visual analog scale (baseline values acu 41 +/- 32, physiotherapy 52 +/- 22; all values extrapolated from figure)	mean % reduction	not measured?	3-point scale	total pain index	Unclear
Control	physiotherapy	physiotherapy	biobehavioral program	Chinese drugs	Metoprolol	massage & relaxation	iprazochrom and dihydroergotoxi nmesylate
Vote count (quality-related)	0	-2	-1	+2	-1	-2	+2

-2 = control group better than acupuncture (significant)
-1 = control group better than acupuncture (trend)
0 = no difference
1 = acupuncture better than control group (trend)
2 = acupuncture better than control group (significant)

The authors of this review make no attempt to draw conclusions from the results of their vote-counting exercise, leaving it to the reader to do the interpretative work.

The interpretation of the results of any vote-counting exercise is a complex task. According to some methodologists the category with the most studies 'wins' (Clinkenbeard 1991). Similarly, in the context of effectiveness reviews, some commentators argue that the statistical significance category 'containing the largest number of studies represents the direction of the true relationship' (Curlette and Cannella 1985). However, as Suri has pointed out, this approach to synthesis analysis and presentation 'tends to give equal weight to studies with different sample sizes and effect sizes at varying significance levels, resulting in misleading conclusions' (Suri 2000), So it is worth being acutely aware of this limitation of vote counting. In general, it should not be used without being adjusted on the basis of a critical appraisal of the studies included in the synthesis.

Techniques for exploring and displaying relationships

As with the preliminary synthesis, the approach required to explore relationships within and between studies will depend in part on whether the evidence to be synthesized is quantitative, qualitative, or both. In the context of systematic reviews of effectiveness, particular attention will need to be paid to the influence of moderator and/or mediator variables which are explored in more detail below. There is a range of techniques that can help support the exploration of relationships within the data – some of these may be appropriate only for one or other type of data, while others can be used with both qualitative and quantitative data.

Idea webbing and concept maps

Used notably in qualitative approaches, these are visual displays of the main concepts or categories of interest. At their simplest these can be handwritten (see Figure 6.1), taking the form of 'mindmaps' (Buzan 1993), for example, noting down core concepts, and the linkages and relationships between them.

Elsewhere these types of maps are referred to as ideas webs or spider

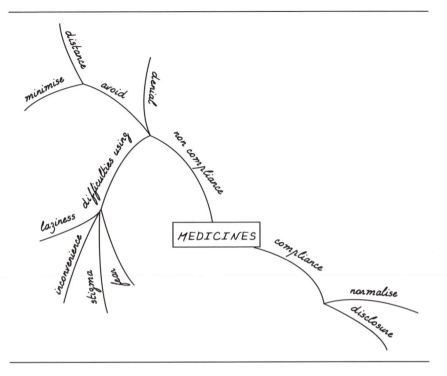

Figure 6.1 'Mindmap' of conceptual ideas on medicine-taking

diagrams (see for example Clinkenbeard 1991 diagram of the connections among the findings reported in the studies included in a review).

More sophisticated versions of this kind of map can be achieved using an organisational chart or a family tree generated by some of the commonly available qualitative data analysis software or word-processing packages. It is also possible to depict different levels of analysis or interpretations with such software and these can be useful when presenting the findings of the synthesis, demonstrating how interpretations were arrived at.

Mulrow et al. (1998) also describe a process of concept mapping – although they do not use this term. Their approach (see Figure 6.2) involves linking multiple pieces of evidence extracted from different studies included in a review to construct a model highlighting the key factors relevant to the review question and representing the relationships between these.

Charts/matrices

Charts, matrices or tables are a commonly used way of displaying qualitative or quantitative information as cells. These can contain numbers/values or

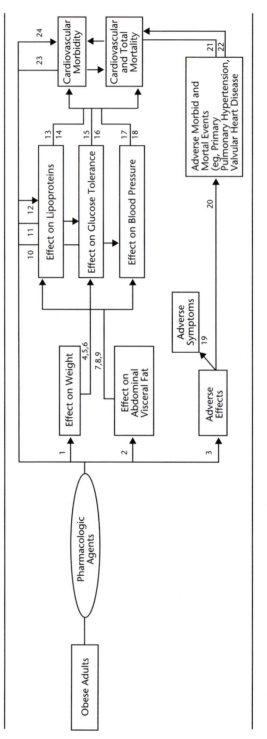

Figure 6.2 An evidence model for the pharmacologic treatment of obesity (Mulrow et al. 1998)

descriptions of variables/concepts. They can be used, as shown in Chapter 4, to compare studies. Simple cross-tabulations can be used, for example, to compare and contrast studies with positive and negative findings for two categories or characteristics. The example in Table 6.4 shows just such a table from an exploratory review of implementation evidence relating to accident prevention initiatives. Here key insights offered by the authors of the primary studies have been extracted from study reports and characterised as 'barriers' and 'facilitators' (similar to the Lloyd Jones example on p. 90 of Chapter 4). These have then been grouped conceptually and presented as a map that synthesizes study findings in such a way that general principles may be read across a number of primary studies. More complex matrices can be used to compare multiple variables or aspects of the studies.

Table 6.4   Identifying Barriers and Facilitators to injury prevention initiatives

Reference	Barriers	Facilitators
Schwarz, DF; Grisso, JA; Miles, C; Holmes, JH and Sutton, RL (1993)	Safety measure requires too much effort from participants' perspectives.	
Ytterstad, B; Smith, GS and Coggan, CA (1998)		Intervention relies on 'passive measures' from the participants' points of view.
Ytterstad, B and Wasmuth, H (1995)	Safety-promoting information is produced but never gets distributed to target groups.	Private companies support the injury-prevention initiative by offering free of low-cost safety products.
Klassen, TP, Mackay, JM; Moher, D, Walker, A and Jones, AL (2000)		Ensuring that interventions are culturally appropriate. Involving the community in the intervention. Not reducing educational interventions to didactic methods. Using a variety of approaches within any one programme of intervention.
Svanström, Leif; Schelp, Lothar; Ekman; Robert and Lindström, Åke (1996).		Community-wide interventions work optimally when the idea comes from within the community.

(continued overleaf)

Table 6.4 *(continued)*

Reference	Barriers	Facilitators
Ekman, Robert and Welander, Glenn (1998)		Ensuring political and intersectoral support. Ensuring optimal distribution of information via the media. Getting support from key political and local figures. Working with a relatively simple, definable focus. Feedback of results maintain the motivation of people engaged in carrying out a programme.

Graphical and statistical presentations

Charts and matrices can be used to present either qualitative or quantitative information. Other means of displaying numerical data include simple displays of counts or frequency distributions. These may be used for content analyses applied to primary qualitative information or for quantitative research. Other techniques commonly used in statistical analyses such as tree plots and funnel displays (Box 6.2) and charts (Figure 6.3) depicting time trends can be used to display large amounts of information relatively economically.

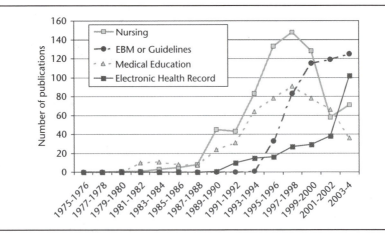

Figure 6.3 Time trend in papers (Greenhalgh 2005 et al.)

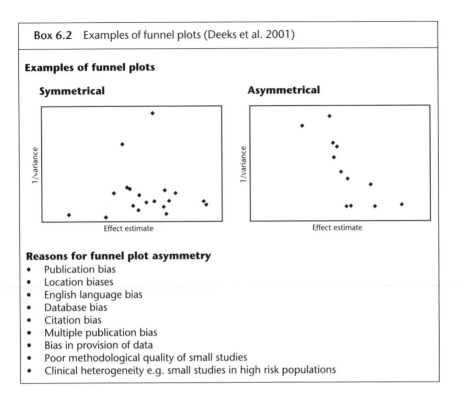

Box 6.2   Examples of funnel plots (Deeks et al. 2001)

Examples of funnel plots

Reasons for funnel plot asymmetry
- Publication bias
- Location biases
- English language bias
- Database bias
- Citation bias
- Multiple publication bias
- Bias in provision of data
- Poor methodological quality of small studies
- Clinical heterogeneity e.g. small studies in high risk populations

Another way of presenting a considerable amount of evidence from a synthesis are Kiviat diagrams (Figure 6.4), sometimes known as radar charts. These display the values of a set of variables (e.g. different dimensions of outcome experienced by a group of service users, or the different impacts of a particular policy) generated by units of interest (e.g. different groups of service users, different interventions or different institutions) on separate axes intersecting at a central point. The values on each spoke can then be joined by lines thereby creating a visual profile of each unit of interest. Where the spokes represent commensurate variables, the area within the joined up points on each spoke can be measured and compared for each member of the population of interest. so, if the variables represented aspects of organisational performance, the organisation with the largest area would be the one with the best overall performance. This sort of plot is used extensively to compare the performance of organisations such as hospitals and clinics, or even entire countries, against one another and in relation to a 'benchmark' (e.g. an average or an ideal level) since a large amount of information can be compressed into a simple diagram. Each organisation can be represented in a different colour and overlaid on national, regional and other average profiles for comparative analysis.

Figure 6.4 charts the relative performance of four different ways of organising primary health care on eight distinct dimensions of performance of interest to health care policy-makers. The data on each aspect of performance and the ratings of each primary health care model were derived from an evidence synthesis designed to feed into primary health care policy development in Canada (Lamarche et al. 2003). The evidence synthesis comprised aggregating qualitative and quantitative research data with data from a Delphi consensus exercise as well as routine information. Note that in this case the outer limits of the diagram are described in terms of 'optimal performance' on each performance variable so that each model can not only be compared with the other three, but also in terms of an ideal primary health care system. From this it can be seen easily that each model has a distinctive performance profile and that some major patterns are easily visible. For example, the two professionally led models are marked by higher accessibility and responsiveness to individual patient demand than the two community-organised models which score more highly on dimensions such as effectiveness, quality and continuity. It is also possible to see that the four models diverge furthest from 'ideal' performance in terms of the 'access' dimension which was seen at the time as a major concern in Canada.

Kiviat or radar charts are relatively easy to produce in that most spreadsheet software packages have a drawing facility. For example, they can be generated in Microsoft Excel 2000 and 2002 as well as Microsoft Office Excel 2003 using the Chart Wizard or the Chart Type command to alter an existing chart created in a different style (e.g. with the data in a table).

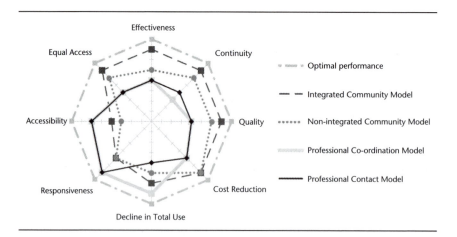

Figure 6.4 Kiviat diagram of the performance of four organisational models of primary health care (Lamarche et al. 2003)

Techniques for displaying the product of the synthesis

Often maps and charts can be developed into diagrams or models that are useful in the presentation of the final synthesis results in a highly condensed form (as opposed to using lengthy narratives). Some can be relatively simple; for example, the model developed from a meta-ethnography of qualitative studies of people with diabetes (Figure 6.5). This depicts a line of argument from a meta-ethnography of seven studies of patients' experiences of diabetes and diabetes care (Campbell et al. 2003). The model suggests that people with diabetes face a number of obstacles and critical stages that they have to overcome to achieve 'balance' or control over the disease (these are depicted in the outer circles in the model). The model does not seek to suggest that people follow identical or linear trajectories, or that they go through the stages/obstacles in any particular order. Rather it shows the key factors that contribute to patients' abilities to cope with their diabetes. The large central oval shows a further element in the line of argument, namely that 'reaching a balance' was closely associated with 'strategic non-compliance' a way of managing the disease 'involving the monitoring and observation of symptoms and an ability to manipulate dietary and medication regimens in order to live life as fully as possible, rather than limiting social and work activities in order to adhere rigidly to medical advice.' (Campbell et al. 2003: 681)

A more complex model is shown in Figure 6.6. This depicts the conceptual model developed from a 'meta-narrative' review of research on organisational innovation (Greenhalgh et al. 2004b, also described in Chapter 1). This model

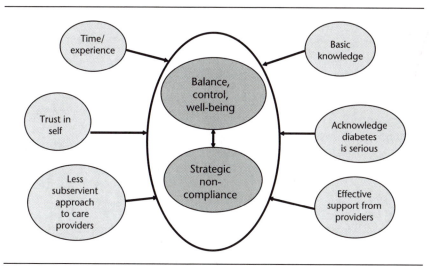

Figure 6.5   Reaching a balance in the management of diabetes (Campbell et al. 2002)

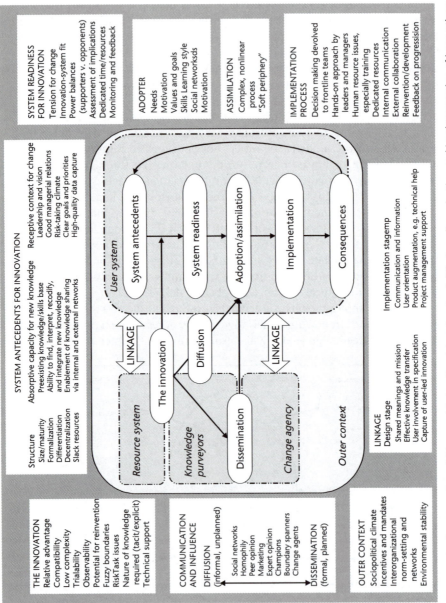

SYSTEM READINESS FOR INNOVATION
Tension for change
Innovation-system fit
Power balances
(supporters v. opponents)
Assessment of implications
Dedicated time/resources
Monitoring and feedback

ADOPTER
Needs
Motivation
Values and goals
Skills Learning style
Social networksds
Motivation

ASSIMILATION
Complex, nonlinear process
"Soft periphery"

IMPLEMENTATION PROCESS
Decision making devolved to frontline teams
Hands-on approach by leaders and managers
Human resource issues, especially training
Dedicated resources
Internal communication
External collaboration
Reinvention/development
Feedback on progression

SYSTEM ANTECEDENTS FOR INNOVATION

Absorptive capacity for new knowledge
Preexisting knowledge/skills base
Ability to find, interpret, recodify, and integrate new knowledge
Enablement of knowledge sharing via internal and external networks

Receptive context for change
Leadership and vision
Good managerial relations
Risk-taking climate
Clear goals and priorities
High-quality data capture

Structure
Size/maturity
Formalization
Differentiation
Decentralization
Slack resources

Implementation stagemp
Communication and information
User orientation
Product augmentation, e.g. technical help
Project management support

LINKAGE
Design stage
Shared meanings and mission
Effective knowledge transfer
User involvement in specification
Capture of user-led innovation

THE INNOVATION
Relative advantage
Compatibility
Low complexity
Trialability
Observability
Potential for reinvention
Fuzzy boundaries
RiskTask issues
Nature of knowledge required (tacit/explicit)
Technical support

COMMUNICATION AND INFLUENCE
DIFFUSION
(informal, unplanned)
Social networks
Homophily
Peer opinion
Marketing
Expert opinion
Champions
Boundary spanners
Change agents
DISSEMINATION
(formal, planned)

OUTER CONTEXT
Sociopolitical climate
Incentives and mandates
Interorganizational norm-setting and networks
Environmental stability

Figure 6.6 Conceptual model for considering the determinants of diffusion, dissemination and implementation of innovations (Greenhalgh et al. 2005, by permission of Elsevier)

is designed to provide a memory aid, showing the principal findings of the review and the complex interactions between them. It is supported, in their paper, by detailed commentary about these findings. In this model the nine boxes of text around the edge of the diagram show the key components identified from the review of nearly 495 sources of research evidence. The main features of the nine components are briefly summarised (e.g. the innnovation needs to offer relative advantage, compatibility, low complexity and so on). In the centre of the diagram the large box depicts the complex relationships and interactions that underpin organisational innovation. For example, there are interrelationships between 'The innovation' and the underlying 'Resource system', the 'Outer context' (i.e. environment) and agents such as 'Knowledge purveyors' and 'Users'. The adoption of the innovation is mediated by how it is diffused, but also by the nature of the user system (e.g. antecedents, readiness and so on).

Software to support synthesis and reviewing

Computer software can be used to support the synthesis process by allowing data storage, retrieval, manipulation and analysis. Some software has the further advantage of allowing the creation of different types of display of the synthesis results.

Many of the commonly used software packages for word-processing, database management and statistic can be used to create the kinds of chart and visual display of the synthesis already described in this chapter. In addition there are a number of software packages designed specifically to support synthesis and/or reviewing. There are various commercial packages designed for qualitative data analysis which could potentially be used to support qualitative synthesis. Each of the packages mentioned below has various organisational chart and pictorial data linkage facilities which can be used when presenting the process or findings of a synthesis.

QSR software and Atlas-Ti

QSR produce software designed to help access, manage and analyse textual and/or multimedia data. Their NUD*IST software now called N6 was developed to support social research and allows qualitative data to be indexed and searched, and has components which can be used to support the generation of theory. QSR also market NVivo7 which also allows coding, retrieval and linking of data. In 2005 QSR released XSight which was designed for market research but potentially would allow the storage, searching and comparison of evidence for synthesis. Atlas-Ti is a similar software package developed by Tom Muhr which offers tools for the systematic qualitative analysis of large bodies of textual, graphical, audio and video data. It assists with selecting, coding, annotating, comparing and synthesizing data. Both these software packages are useful for organising data during the synthesis process and they have facilities to print output (such as organisational charts and spider diagrams).

Although these packages have a longer history of use in primary research, they could potentially be used to support synthesis. One of the few examples of the use of such software in mixed qualitative and quantitative synthesis is the interpretive approach used by Dixon-Woods and colleagues (2006b). In this synthesis of qualitative and quantitative research evidence on access to health care, all the data were transformed into text, QSR N5 was used to facilitate the identification of themes and a comparative analysis was then undertaken.

RevMan

RevMan is the Cochrane Collaboration's program for preparing and maintaining Cochrane reviews (see www.cc-ims.net/RevMan). It was developed by the Nordic Cochrane Centre and is overseen by the Information Management System Group (IMSG) and the RevMan Advisory Group of the Cochrane Collaboration. RevMan can be used to enter protocols, as well as complete reviews, including text, characteristics of studies, comparison tables and study data. It can perform meta-analysis of the data entered, and present the results graphically.

JBI-CReMS, SUMARI and QARI

A team of academics at the Joanna Briggs Institute, in Adelaide, Australia is developing a software package called SUMARI designed to assist health and other researchers and practitioners to conduct systematic reviews (see http:// www.joannabriggs.edu.au/services/sumari.php). This software package consists of five modules. The core module is the Comprehensive Review Management System (JBI-CReMS) which allows reviewers not only to follow the standard approach developed by the Cochrane Collaboration, but also to incorporate other forms of evidence using additional SUMARI modules. The Qualitative Assessment and Review Instrument (JBI-QARI) module is designed to manage, appraise, analyse and synthesize textual (qualitative) data as part of a systematic review. It is web-based and incorporates a critical appraisal scale; data extraction forms; a data synthesis function; and a reporting function. There are also plans to develop a module for Narrative, Opinion and Text Assessment and Review Instrument (JBI-NOTARI) which will allow the incorporation of expert opinion and other textual material.

Issues of style and voice

The style and language used to present synthesis findings has to be accessible to the target audience or audiences. This will mean paying attention to the language, notably the use of jargon or terminology, but will also affect the level of complexity in the reporting. Some funders require that research reports conform to particular conventions. Others require that reports are written in a style and language accessible to particular groups, for example following the principles developed by the Plain English Campaign (http://www.plainenglish.co.uk). Reports, and in particular journal papers, may have restrictions on word length and it is therefore necessary to make decisions about how much detail can be provided. Often journals will require that tables summarising included and excluded studies be made available separately on websites since systematic reviews can be cumbersome to present in full in journal format.

It is worth paying attention to the issue of how ideas are conveyed through writing and presentation. As van Maanen points out, writing requires 'decisions about what to tell and how to tell it' (1988: 25). At a basic level it may be worth considering whether to use the first or third person, and an active or passive voice in presenting the synthesis, as well as how much information to provide about the background, experience and possible biases of the review team. In primary qualitative research, particularly, the question of whether to let the participants or subjects of research 'speak for themselves' or whether to impose the researchers' interpretations when presenting the findings is often encountered. Reports and presentations of the research usually try to balance these twin demands. Synthesis introduces an additional level of complexity in the interpretation or analysis – for example, a synthesis of published research evidence needs to represent the participants of the individual studies included in the synthesis, the interpretations and findings offered by the authors of those studies, *and* the cumulative interpretations and results of the synthesis.

Reports

Often one of the key reasons for disseminating the results of a synthesis is to meet the conditions or expectations of funders. Many funding bodies have standardised reporting methods and formats and sometimes it can be quite a challenge to produce the results of a synthesis in a way that meets these requirements.

It is thus important to keep the audience and funders' requirements in mind during the writing up. The synthesis will usually produce a large amount of material. While policy-makers and advisors may require some detail and description of arguments, politicians are likely to want only a single page, and no more, summarising the synthesis. These policy and political audiences may not be interested in the process of the synthesis (except to be assured that 'good practice' has been adhered to) and may not, therefore, require full descriptions of methods or theoretical positions adopted by the researchers. Other audiences of reviews and synthesis may require these details, and from the point of view of transparency (see below) it is important that these details are available when required, for example, in appendices or separate documents on a website.

The exact structure and format of written reports of synthesis will depend on the audience and any requirements from funders and commissioners. It is usual to report what the synthesis has found and account for the methods and studies included. A suggested generic structure is given below.

Summary

Ideally this needs to be kept short and to the point. Some audiences will not require more than a page and sometimes a paragraph will suffice. Longer executive summaries should really not go over 2–3 pages maximum. It can be helpful to focus the reader on the key messages of the synthesis and what insights integrating the studies yielded.

Background

Depending on the length of the overall report it can be helpful to locate the synthesis findings in some wider context. Mention can be made of any previous reviews and/or the rationale for conducting the synthesis. It is worth noting the applicability and scope of the synthesis, for example, whether the evidence included is national or international, and whether the synthesis is designed for a policy or research audience, and/or for decision or knowledge support.

Questions /aims

This should detail the overall question or aims and any sub-questions or adaptations made as the synthesis progressed.

Methods

This should describe the methods in sufficient detail for the reader to judge validity and credibility. This means reporting on aspects such as search strategy, selection criteria, quality appraisal (if used), data extraction, the methods used for the synthesis and their justifications.

Findings

This should contain the results of the synthesis with supporting evidence and argument from the individual studies and the analysis where necessary, including the relationship between the original findings, the interpretations of the primary researchers and the interpretations advanced by the synthesis. It should explore any heterogeneity between the findings of individual studies.

Discussion/recommendations and conclusions
This includes the interpretation of the findings and potential application to problems or other settings. It is often wise to include some consideration of the strengths and weaknesses of the methods and results. Most reports will also include some discussion of the practical implications of these findings for policy or management.

Technical appendices
These can include full details of the search strategy and the results of the searches, a full bibliography including all the studies included and excluded, and details of the findings of each of the included studies. This can also be the place to put details of any quality appraisal process, depending on the audience for the report.

Journal papers and oral presentations

These may be condensed versions of longer reports made to funding bodies or sponsors. They need to cover much the same ground as the written report, but may be required to do so much more succinctly – either in terms of word limits or time allowed to present.

For conference reports and other oral presentations the key is timing; it is worth working out exactly how much time is available for the presentation and ensuring that material fits within these time constraints (see the 'lift pitch' in Box 6.3 as an example of how to focus a presentation). Often it may only be possible to get one or two main messages from the synthesis across. A presentation to a policy audience – for example chief executives of health care organisations – may require a different structure from an academic presentation. It is likely that senior managers will not warm to a detailed description of the

---

Box 6.3   The lift (elevator) pitch

One trick for thinking about summarising the results of a synthesis (or indeed any research) is the idea of the lift 'pitch'. Imagine that you have entered a lift (elevator) with the person who is the audience for your report. You have the time it takes for the lift to travel three floors to explain your results.

Thinking like this can help focus the mind on what are the key messages you need to get across.

methods used, but this would be expected by researchers. There are limits to the detail that can be absorbed in this kind of presentation and to the attention span of the audience. To manage this, it is helpful to stick to a few key points and where possible provide illustrations (e.g. graphs, concept maps, flow charts, spider diagrams, etc.) which support these. An oral presentation can be supported by information about where to obtain more detailed material, so brief handouts/ summaries or details of a website for further information are helpful.

Web reports

Increasingly research reports and other materials are disseminated via the World Wide Web. However, there is a tendency to use the large storage power of the web simply to house written reports such as the final reports or copies of publications rather than harnessing the potential of this format. Of course the capacity of the web to make long documents available and relatively easy to access does mean that it is useful as an archive of longer reports and technical appendices. However in terms of dissemination to policy- and decision-makers, this format for all its accessibility may not be that useful. It may therefore be worth thinking about using some of the features of information technology – such as hyperlinks and signposting – which allow the reader to navigate through these materials more readily, so that different readers can choose which parts of the overall project output they wish to scan and which to avoid. This can be particularly helpful in producing flexible outputs which are relevant to different audiences. Essentially the reader can choose what information and how much she or he wants to take in.

Reports for policy- and decision-makers

Reports for policy- and decision-makers are likely to be different to the kinds of output associated with academic reporting, such as journal papers. Policy and management reports need, above all to be succinct and targeted at an audience, most of whom have a limited amount of time to read and who are often involved in fast-moving decision processes.

The Canadian Health Services Research Foundation (CHSRF) has pioneered what they refer to as Reader-Friendly Writing and a format which they call '1:3:25'. As well as being used extensively in Canada, this format is also recommended and is gaining currency elsewhere. The CHSRF is clear that: 'Writing a research summary for decision-makers is not the same as writing an article for an academic journal. It has a different objective, and it takes a different approach.' The idea of a 1:3:25 report is that page 1 contains just the main messages, this is followed by a three-page executive summary and then a

25-page maximum presentation of the findings 'in language a bright educated, but not research-trained person would understand' (see Box 6.4).

The Synthesis Project is an initiative of The Robert Wood Johnson Foundation (RWJF) to produce concise and thought-provoking briefs and reports that translate reviews of research findings on perennial health policy questions into accessible formats (http://www.rwjf.org/publications/synthesis/about-_the_project/index.html). Synthesis products are tailored to the diverse needs of policy-makers and analysts, and include both 'policy briefs', namely short and skimmable summaries highlighting major findings and policy implications, and longer 'synthesis reports' that provide more in-depth and layered information, plus analysis of information gaps and questions for future research. The RWJF also makes extensive use of charts as ways of providing data and information sources within policy briefs and research synthesis reports. An example of a RWJF policy brief is found in Box 6.5 (page 144).

Box 6.4 Reader-Friendly Writing (CHSRF, www.chsrf.ca)

The Canadian Health Services Research Foundation has a mandate to fund a different kind of research – practically oriented work done in collaboration with the people who run the healthcare system, to answer their very concrete questions about how to make the system work better. That means a different style of writing for your final report.
inference – how well is this explained?

Writing a research summary for decision makers is not the same as writing an article for an academic journal. It has a different objective, and it takes a different approach.

1:3:25

Every report prepared for the foundation has the same guidelines: start with one page of main messages; follow that with a three-page executive summary; present your findings in no more than 25 pages of writing, in language a bright, educated, but not research-trained person would understand.

Main Messages

The one in the foundation's 1:3:25 rule is one page of main message bullets. They are the heart of your report, the lessons decision makers can take from your research. Don't confuse them with a summary of findings: you have to go one step further and tell your audience what you think the findings mean for them. The messages, per se, may not even appear in the text. They are what can be inferred from your report. This is your chance, based on your research, to tell decision makers what implications your work has for theirs.

How to formulate them? Set aside your text and focus on expressing clear conclusions based on what you've learned. Consider your audience – who are they, and what do they most need to know about what you've learned? Summon up that bright, educated reader and answer this question for him or her: So what does this really *mean*?

(continued overleaf)

Box 6.4 (continued)

Say your study is on how to set budgets in a regional health system. You've found a tendency to keep money flowing on traditional lines. That's the problem. The actual main message you write may be that it's wiser to focus on reallocating other resources – people, space, equipment – to health promotion than to take cash away from acute care.

A study on the impact of increasing use of homecare might show that hip-implant patients regain mobility faster out of hospital than as inpatients. The key message would be to encourage early discharge. Spell it out.

Your study has found that job security is the biggest factor driving nurses to work in the U.S. Your main message might be that governments should make 10-year commitments to funding levels for nursing services.

Writing main messages can be difficult for researchers to do, trained as they are to be detached and to collect evidence, rather than judge it, but it has to be done if research is to be of real use to decision makers. And remember – if you don't do it, you're leaving your work to be interpreted by someone else, who won't likely have your insight.

This is not to say that you have to come up with definitive recommendations from research that just doesn't offer them. Be as concrete as you can and then, if you're really not ready to draw more conclusions, don't just fall back on 'more research is needed.' Use your main messages to define the questions that still need to be asked.

Executive Summary

The three in 1:3:25 is the executive summary. These are your findings condensed to serve the needs of the busy decision maker, who wants to know quickly whether the report will be useful.

Start by outlining what issues you were looking at, using language and examples a local hospital administrator or ministry official will understand; sum up the answers you found. An executive summary is not an academic abstract; it's much more like a newspaper story, where the most interesting stuff goes at the top, followed by the background and context and less important information further down. This is not the place for more than a line or two about your approach, methods and other technical details. Concentrate on getting the essence of your research across succinctly but not cryptically.

The Report

The foundation allots 25 pages for the complete report of your work (double-spaced with 12-point type and 2.5 cm margins). This may be a length you're more comfortable with, but don't lapse into academic style just because you have more room. Don't hesitate to use anecdotes or stories to get your point across. To make sure your writing suits the busy decision maker, intelligent and interested, but not an academic, take the time to show it to your decision-maker partners. What do they find most useful and interesting? How do they find your language and style? As a guide, the foundation has set seven categories that must be covered in the report, in the order given:

Context: outline the policy issue or managerial problem your research addresses. State the research question clearly. Highlight earlier research and the contribution current research may make. Anecdotes can work well here.

Implications: State what your findings mean for decision makers. Note what different types of audiences may be interested in your work, and if the research has different messages for those different audiences, separate and label them. Notes on how broadly the information can be generalized should go here. This is where the essence of your key messages is found.

Approach: Outline your methods, including the design of the study, the sources of data and details on the sample, the response rate and analysis techniques. Describe how you worked with decision makers on the project, and outline your plans for dissemination. Highly technical material can be an appendix: here you should focus on explaining why these details matter, how they might affect the study results and conclusions and why you chose one approach over another.

Results: Summarize your results to show how they support the conclusions you have presented, highlighting

themes and messages. Use graphs and tables if they will improve understanding. Results that don't relate directly to the conclusions should be moved to an appendix.

Additional Resources: Not for other researchers – although they may find it useful – this is the place to give information on publications, web sites and other useful sources of information for decision makers.

Further Research: Outline gaps in knowledge; frame questions on management and policy issues you've identified and suggest studies to answer them.

References and Bibliography: References in the report should use consecutive superscript numbering and be presented as endnotes, not in the body of the text or the foot of the page. The bibliography should highlight those items most useful for decision makers and researchers wanting to do more reading and also include useful reading beyond that used in the report, including some easy-to-read pieces to give decision makers background. The references and bibliography count as part of the report's 25 pages, unless they are fully annotated, in which case they can be put into an appendix.

Box 6.5 Example A of a RWJF Policy Brief (www.rwjf.org/publications/synthesis/reports-and-briefs/pdf/no6_policybrief.pdf)

Geographic variation in Medicare per capita spending: Should policy-makers be concerned?

Claudia H. Williams and Marsha Gold, Sc.D., based on a Research Synthesis by Marsha Gold.

SUMMARY OF KEY FINDINGS

> **More than half the variation in Medicare spending is due to geographic differences in health care utilization.** Price and population differences account for less than half the variation.

> **People living in areas with more hospitals and doctors relative to population receive more services.** Yet we still don't know much about why practices vary so greatly across areas.

> **Higher spending is not associated with better care.** People in higher spending areas use more services but do not have more appropriate care, better health outcomes, or reduced mortality.

Why is this issue relevant to today's policy debates?

▦ In contrast to the uniformity of benefits and eligibility, Medicare spending varies geographically. This leads to the sense that some providers and beneficiaries "win"—receiving more services, higher revenues, better benefits—and some "lose." Concern over these disparities has fueled Medicare policy debates.

▦ This brief analyzes reasons for geographic variation in Medicare spending per capita, identifies what factors—including differences in population characteristics, prices, and patterns of care—account for these variations, and discusses the policy implications of these findings.

Does Medicare spending vary geographically?

▦ Medicare per capita spending varies widely and persistently by area.

In 1996, spending per capita in the highest spending area ($8,500) was almost three times as high as spending in the lowest ($3,000). Only about one-third of regions had spending within 10 percent of the average (Figure 1).

Figure 1. Unadjusted Medicare spending per beneficiary, 1996

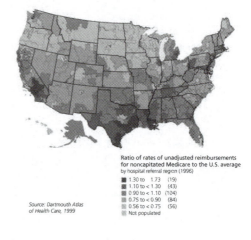

Source: Dartmouth Atlas of Health Care, 1999

Ratio of rates of unadjusted reimbursements for noncapitated Medicare to the U.S. average by hospital referral region (1996)
- 1.30 to 1.73 (19)
- 1.10 to < 1.30 (43)
- 0.90 to < 1.10 (104)
- 0.75 to < 0.90 (84)
- 0.56 to < 0.75 (56)
- Not populated

▦ There are three potential reasons for geographic spending variation: differences across areas in population characteristics; differences in price; and differences in service.

Box 6.5 (continued)

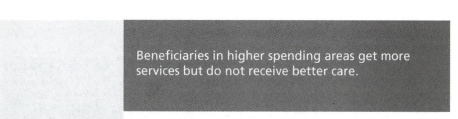

Beneficiaries in higher spending areas get more
services but do not receive better care.

Use varies across areas because
of differences in:

— Supply of services
— Provider training
— Provider preferences
— Patient demand

While research documents a strong
positive relationship between the
supply of services and their use, it
provides limited insights on why
practices vary so much across the
country and how to reduce this
variation.

People in higher spending areas
get more, but not necessarily
better care. One study examining
outcomes of care for colorectal
cancer, acute myocardial infarction
and hip fracture found that
people in higher spending regions
received 60 percent more care,
but did not have better mortality
rates, functional status or higher
satisfaction.

How much of the variation is due to differences in population mix and prices across areas?

▮ While estimates vary, most studies show that population and price differences
account for less than half the variation in per capita Medicare spending by
region. One study found that adjusting for these factors (Figure 2) reduced
spending variation by only about 18 percent.

Figure 2. Medicare spending variation before and after adjusting for population
and price differences, 1996*

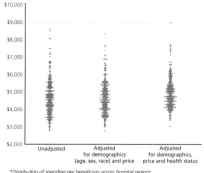

*Distribution of spending per beneficiary across hospital regions
Source: Dartmouth Atlas of Health Care, 1999

▮ Because population and certain influences on price (e.g., wage levels) are not
under the control of the delivery system or policy-makers, comparisons of per
capita spending are usually adjusted for them.

What explains the remaining variation?

▮ The remaining variation is explained by differences in the use of health care
services across areas including the number, mix, intensity and setting of services.
These factors account for more than half the variation in spending.

Do people in higher spending (i.e., higher use) areas get better care?

▮ Beneficiaries in higher spending areas use more services but do not seem to
receive better care or to have superior health outcomes. Indeed, some studies
show lower quality of care in states where beneficiaries use more services.

▮ In both high- and low-spending areas, however, beneficiaries receive
inappropriate care, involving overuse, underuse and misuse of services.

Box 6.5 (continued)

Policy Implications

REFERENCES

Figure 1: J.E. Wennberg et al. *The Dartmouth Atlas of Health Care in the United States.* AHA Press: Dartmouth Medical School. Center for Evaluative Clinical Sciences, 1999.

Figure 2: M. Gold. *Geographic differences in Medicare per capita spending: Should policy-makers be concerned?* Research Synthesis Report, the Synthesis Project, 2004.

Figure 3: Wennberg, 1999.

> **Some causes of variation are more amenable to policy intervention than others.** Population characteristics, for example, are generally immutable, whereas other sources of variation such as price and service use might be affected by policy.

> **Because differences in patterns of use, and not prices, explain most of the variation in spending, changes in administered prices (for fee-for-service Medicare) will not make spending much more uniform.**

> **While higher spending is not associated with better health care, simply reducing spending in higher cost areas will not produce more effective and efficient care.** Evidence-based medicine might produce more effective care, but will not guarantee savings because some services will be used less but others will be used more.

> **Rather than focusing on spending variation per se, Medicare could concentrate on rewarding quality.** Approaches might include support for centers of excellence, payment systems that reward quality, and promotion of disease management for high-cost users.

> **Geographic variation in spending will not go away if Medicare moves to a more competitive model.** Even under competitive bidding, capitation rates will likely reflect differences in prices and medical practice across the country.

> **This issue is bigger than Medicare.** Although data are lacking, the same geographic variation in spending that exists in Medicare is likely to occur among other payers and populations. Policy-makers might consider what responsibility to assume for measuring or modifying such differences.

There are other examples of ways of presenting research findings for policy audiences, and whilst these have not all been directly linked to synthesis they do provide templates for how one might communicate reviews in the context of policy and management decision-making. A similar format to that used by RWJF is used by the Joseph Rowntree Foundation for their 'Findings' briefings which are part of a larger strategy for disseminating research output. One feature of the 'Findings' reports is that they are available in different formats; for example, the web-based version makes extensive use of hyperlinks to allow access to longer material and supporting documents (see Box 6.6).

As with the other types of presentation discussed in this chapter it is important to consider engaging with the audience for reports to policy- and decision-makers earlier rather than later in the synthesis process. For these audiences it is especially important to provide a clear summary even if the messages are about the uncertainty of the current stage of knowledge. It may also be important to follow up any written reporting with face-to-face discussions with the decision-makers involved (see Chapter 7).

Specific issues in reporting qualitative synthesis

Within the qualitative research community there has long been a recognition that writing and presentation of qualitative research is about representing the data and that this representation is influenced by the theoretical and methodological stance of the researcher. Writing up qualitative research needs to be at once coherent, but also to capture the richness of qualitative data. White et al. note that this is a real challenge because it is not easy to summarise qualitative findings neatly, say by presenting tables or numbers. Qualitative researchers, therefore, have to find ways to order 'disorderly data' (White et al. 2003: 289). The same issues confront those engaged in synthesizing qualitative research – either alone or with quantitative research evidence. For a synthesis involving any qualitative evidence, a further problem for some of the potential audiences may be a lack of familiarity with qualitative research methods. It is therefore important that in presenting the findings the reader is made aware of the types of study included and the kinds of inference and interpretation that are possible.

A frequent criticism of qualitative research is that its method of analysis is something of a 'black box' (Kvale 1996) and that qualitative researchers need to get better at explaining why methods were chosen and how results were arrived at. Again this also applies to a synthesis involving qualitative evidence – it is important to be clear about which methods were chosen and why (see Chapter 8 for more on this), and to be as transparent as possible in detailing how findings were arrived at.

Box 6.6   Example of JRF 'findings' (www.jrf.org.UK/knowledge/findings/socialcare/
1959.asp)

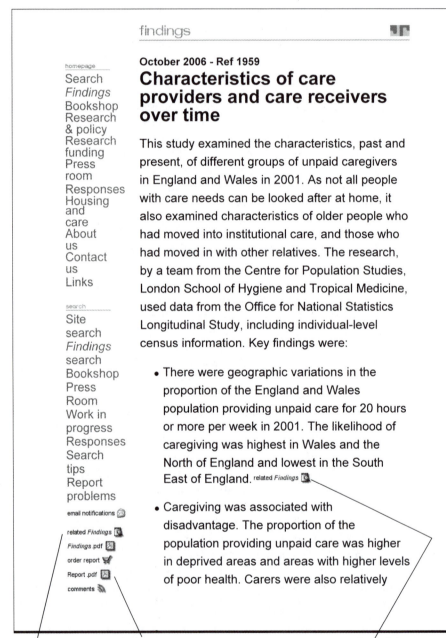

findings

homepage
Search
Findings
Bookshop
Research
& policy
Research
funding
Press
room
Responses
Housing
and
care
About
us
Contact
us
Links

search
Site
search
Findings
search
Bookshop
Press
Room
Work in
progress
Responses
Search
tips
Report
problems

email notifications

related *Findings*

Findings .pdf

order report

Report .pdf

comments

October 2006 - Ref 1959

Characteristics of care providers and care receivers over time

This study examined the characteristics, past and present, of different groups of unpaid caregivers in England and Wales in 2001. As not all people with care needs can be looked after at home, it also examined characteristics of older people who had moved into institutional care, and those who had moved in with other relatives. The research, by a team from the Centre for Population Studies, London School of Hygiene and Tropical Medicine, used data from the Office for National Statistics Longitudinal Study, including individual-level census information. Key findings were:

- There were geographic variations in the proportion of the England and Wales population providing unpaid care for 20 hours or more per week in 2001. The likelihood of caregiving was highest in Wales and the North of England and lowest in the South East of England. related *Findings*

- Caregiving was associated with disadvantage. The proportion of the population providing unpaid care was higher in deprived areas and areas with higher levels of poor health. Carers were also relatively

summary   longer
report   hyperlink

disadvantaged and more likely than others of the same age to be in poor health themselves. related *Findings*

- Those from Bangladeshi and Pakistani ethnic groups were more likely to provide care than those from other ethnic groups, once age profile and gender were taken into account. related *Findings*

- Caregivers were less likely than others of the same age to be employed. Among those who were employed, women working in the public sector were more likely than those in the private sector to be carers. Women who had worked in a caring profession were more likely to become unpaid carers. related *Findings*

- Some 9 per cent of women and 4 per cent of men aged 65 and over and living in the community in 1991 were in institutional care by 2001. These proportions were slightly lower than the equivalent between 1981 and 1991. Characteristics associated with increased chances of moving into institutional care included older age, being unmarried, poorer health, being a tenant rather than an owner occupier and, among women, having no children. related *Findings*

Qualitative-quantitative synthesis

Careful consideration should be given to the particular issues surrounding the presentation of a synthesis of qualitative with quantitative research evidence. One model is to have two distinct syntheses (e.g. a statistical meta-analysis and qualitative meta-ethnography) and to present these separately followed by a discussion which seeks to integrate the two sets of conclusions. The EPPI centre has developed this model (see Chapter 5) and undertaken a slightly more sophisticated integration of two distinct syntheses using some of the matrix/charting approaches described earlier (Figure 6.7).

The presentation of the synthesis needs to make clear which sources contributed which findings. It is worth considering how the qualitative and quantitative findings are related; for example, does the qualitative analysis extend or explain the quantitative evidence, or vice versa? This can inform the sequence of reporting in a report. There is also a need to consider the possibility of conflicting findings and decide how these will be dealt with.

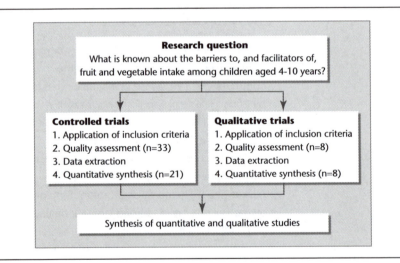

Figure 6.7 Stages of the review (Thomas et al. 2004)

Transparency

Rigorous synthesis and reviewing means that research must be presented in ways that enable scrutiny. The demands of rigour mean that the reader can follow what was done and how conclusions were arrived at. An audit trail should describe the process of analysis in enough detail so that readers can follow how interpretations or conclusions derived from synthesis were arrived at. This means providing a clear account of methods to display credibility.

A key feature of systematic reviews is that they aim for reproducibility. This may be less attainable in qualitative synthesis, but still worth striving for. Van Maanen (1988), writing about ethnography, suggests that researchers construct different types of tale about their research. Interpretive-based syntheses may not be reproducible in the sense that they arrive at exactly the same conclusions irrespective of who undertakes them. Dixon-Woods et al. make this same point, recognising that 'alternative accounts of the same evidence might be possible using different authorial voices' and go on to emphasise, however, that 'all accounts should be grounded in the evidence, verifiable and plausible, and that reflexivity will be a paramount requirement' (2006a: 39). This is as much as any account can reasonably achieve. There can be no absolute requirement for all analysts to reach exactly the same conclusions.

Resources for presenting the results of a synthesis

This chapter has provided some ideas about different ways of presenting the results of a synthesis. How many of these strategies can be employed is largely a question of resources and time. There may also be limits in terms of skills in 'knowledge transfer'. Some research funding bodies such as the NHS Service Delivery and Organisation Research and Development Programme and the Canadian Health Services Research Foundation (CHSRF) have recognised that researchers are not always the best people to present or disseminate their findings in practice and policy settings. They have introduced skilled knowledge brokers and communication experts who are tasked with the job of translating research findings into formats that are more accessible to practitioners and decision-makers (see Chapter 8 for more discussion of 'knowledge transfer'). This may also be appropriate for disseminating and presenting the findings of a synthesis

Summary

Organising findings and presenting them is a vital part of the synthesis process and one which needs to be planned and thought about well in advance of the closing stages of any project or review. Presentations need to be carefully structured and targeted at the potential audience(s). This means finding a clear and accessible way to tell the 'story' of the synthesis utilising whichever reporting formats and styles are appropriate. The presentation of the synthesis is also a core activity for ensuring rigour and quality in the synthesis process. Any presentation needs to provide a transparent account of the process of the review with sufficient detail for the reader to judge its validity and quality.

7 Using evidence reviews for policy- and decision-making

The idea that research should be useful is described by Solesbury (2001) as the 'utilitarian turn' and this view of the role of research is increasingly a feature of the health field. Starting in the late 1980s, the so called 'evidence-based medicine' (EBM) movement came to prominence (Pope 2003). EBM proposes that clinical practice decisions should be based as far as possible on the available research evidence, particularly from randomised controlled trials (RCTs) of the effectiveness of different procedures and treatments. In the latter half of the 1990s, the movement towards evidence-based clinical practice broadened to include the aspiration towards 'evidence-based policy' (see Chapter 1, p. 9). According to its proponents, public policy, including decisions about the financing, organisation and delivery of health services and public health, should be more securely rooted in an understanding of the findings of relevant research and other sources of evidence than they have been in the past. Informed by an awareness of the complexity of policy-making and the limitations of research, other proponents of the greater use of evidence in the policy process prefer to advocate the use of the term 'evidence-informed policy' stressing the integration of experience, judgement and expertise with the best available external evidence from systematic research (Davies 1999) rather than evidence directly determining policy. Increasingly too, research funders expect research findings to be 'used' in some way to justify the resources spent, and they require researchers applying for grants to propose strategies for the dissemination and uptake of their findings.

Systematic reviews and evidence-informed policy and management

Despite differences of ambition, all those involved in the various strands of the 'evidence' movement believe that better policy decisions (and presumably better processes and perhaps eventual outcomes) can be achieved if decision-makers have better access to, and make more use of, information, particularly from research, throughout the policy and decision process (i.e. from agenda setting, through policy formulation, implementation and subsequent evaluation). Systematic reviews are seen as particularly helpful in this process because they bring together in one place the findings from many studies and attempt to ascertain what the collected knowledge means to people who do not have the time or expertise to cope with what are often vast and confusing bodies of evidence. It is clear that most public decision-makers are exposed to frequent claims and counter-claims from advocates, interest groups, experts and professional bodies, who typically make use of the best-known or the latest studies to advance their arguments. Sheldon (2005) argues that policy-makers and managers are vulnerable to being misled when they hear about the latest well-publicised study since individual pieces of research frequently suffer from low statistical power (in the case of quantitative studies of effectiveness); are more susceptible to individual researcher bias; provide an incomplete picture, by definition, of an issue; and cannot easily take account of the contextual variability in, say, the impact of an intervention since most will have been conducted in a specific setting. He argues that the policy relevance of individual studies is lowered particularly by the fact that they can rarely identify the factors across settings that modify the costs, benefits and harms of particular policies or programmes. By contrast, systematic reviews are a better source of evidence, in general, for decision-makers, on the grounds that:

- the likelihood of being misled is lower than in the case of single studies (this is especially the case for studies of effectiveness);
- the confidence that can be placed in the findings is greater than with a single study (again, especially if the question is one of effectiveness);
- they enable a more efficient use of time and effort on the part of decision-makers since someone or a group with greater expertise does the hard work of assembling, distilling, weighing, integrating and interpreting the evidence, and this is then brought together in a manageable form;
- they can be more constructively debated and contested than individual studies which can seem to contradict one another in a manner which decision-makers often find frustrating (in other words, it is easier to identify the reasons for heterogeneity in the results of individual studies in the context of a synthesis and, if appropriate, estimate an overall effect size within narrower confidence limits than would be possible in a single study) (Lavis et al. 2005).

The relationship between 'evidence' and 'policy'

In a simplistic model of knowledge (or evidence) transfer, practitioners and decision-makers need only be presented with a review or summary of the evidence to implement its findings. However, it is widely observed that simply disseminating evidence, even when derived from syntheses and presented in an accessible a way (see Chapter 6), is normally insufficient to ensure that it is taken up and used either for policy or practice decision-making. The relationship between evidence (from research or other sources) and decision-making is complex, and has been much studied and debated, particularly in the past decade (Davies et al. 2000; Lin and Gibson 2003), especially in the health field. There is frequently frustration among researchers and advocates of more evidence-influenced or evidence-based decision-making that evidence does not seem to play a sufficiently large role in policy and practice. One of the reasons for this frustration is that advocates' conceptions of how policy and management decisions are made are frequently some version of a rational, linear model in which a problem is identified, a range of possible solutions is located, these are assessed for their relative costs and benefits using the available research evidence, the best solution is chosen and implemented, and the impact of the chosen solution is subsequently evaluated to see if it needs amendment. Under this conception, if there appears to be a problem in the use of evidence, this is usually attributed to a lack of pertinent evidence, a lack of access to the evidence, a lack of expertise to interpret and use evidence, or a lack of understanding among decision-makers of the importance of evidence for informing decision-making. As Lomas puts it, under this model, 'The research-policy arena is assumed to be a retail store in which researchers are busy filling shelves of a shop front with a comprehensive set of all possible studies that a decision-maker might some day drop by to purchase' (2000: 141).

The 'enlightenment' model

In fact, most studies of the use of research evidence in policy and management decisions support a much more indirect notion of the relationship between scientific endeavour and decision-making than the retail store. From a series of classic studies in the USA in the 1970s and 1980s, Weiss concluded that new knowledge and insights from social research appeared to 'percolate' into the various strata of the political environment before being taken up by political actors, much as water falling on limestone is absorbed into the ground, disappears, filters downward through multiple, hard-to-observe channels and then reappears unexpectedly some time later elsewhere in the landscape. She termed this the 'enlightenment' role of research (Weiss 1979; 1986) in which new knowledge 'creeps' in a convoluted, hard-to-predict, way into the consciousness of policy-makers and managers primarily at the level of ideas and broad orientations rather than in the shape of specific bodies of findings or proposals for action. The process was far from the linear, predictable sequence of influencing events described in simple 'rational' models of the way in which research should influence decisions (Table 7.1 summarises the differences between the two models of the relationship). As a result, it was inherently difficult to 'engineer' the use of research evidence by decision-makers.

In further research, Weiss (1991) identified three basic forms of knowledge created by research, generated to some extent by different styles and methods of research:

- data and findings;
- ideas and criticism, emerging from the findings and associated with the 'enlightenment' model of how research influences policy;
- arguments for action, deriving from the findings and the ideas generated by the research and extending the role of the researcher towards advocacy of change.

Each is likely to be seen as useful by potential end-users in different circumstances. For example, data and findings are likely to be associated with a more instrumental use of evidence, whereas ideas and criticism are more likely to contribute to an enlightenment model of use. Weiss argued that apparently

Table 7.1 Differences between the 'engineering' and 'enlightenment' models of how research influences policy (Buse et al. 2005)

Engineering or problem-solving model	Enlightenment model
Sees relationship between research and policy as rational and sequential	Sees relationship as indirect and not necessarily logical or neat
A problem exists because basic research has identified it	Problems are not always recognized, or at least not immediately.
Applied research is undertaken to help solve the problem	There may be a considerable period of time between research and its impact on policy. Much research develops new ways of thinking rather than solutions to specific problems.
Research is then applied to helping solve the policy problem. Research produces a preferred policy solution	The way in which research influences policy is complex and hidden. Policy makers may not want to act on results
Rarely or never describes how the relationship between research and policy works in practice	How research influences policy is indirectly via a 'black box', the functioning of which is hidden from view rather than explained

objective data and findings were likely to have their greatest influence when a clear problem had already been recognised by all actors and where there was consensus about the range of feasible policy responses. In this situation, the role of research was to help decide which response to adopt. Ideas and criticism, by contrast, appeared to be most useful in open, pluralistic policy systems and when there was uncertainty about the nature of the policy or management problem (or even whether there was one worthy of attention), as well as a wide range of possible policy responses available. The third category – research as argument – she identified as most useful when there was a high degree of conflict over an issue and where the implications of the research were promoted in an explicitly political way. In this situation, the impact of the research depended on the advocacy skills of the researchers (or their allies) and whether key policy stakeholders agreed with the values and goals underlying the changes being proposed on the basis of the research findings. Research as argument would only have an influence if researchers took the gamble of abandoning their customary status as disinterested producers of knowledge and entered the unpredictable world of political argument and counter-argument.

Weiss further showed that the most common use of evidence when it did finally occur was not to influence a specific course of action (associated with 'research as argument'), but to help define the policy 'problem' in the first place; for example, changing people's ideas about the nature of a phenomenon so that it was more likely to be seen as a 'problem' and, therefore, a legitimate focus for public policy action (the 'ideas and criticism' form, described above). As Black (2001: 277) puts it, 'Research is considered less as problem solving than as a process of argument or debate to create concern and set the agenda'.

The 'enlightenment' model of the use of research in policy and management decision-making is helpful in highlighting that research evidence (or indeed evidence from other sources) is normally only one of many factors contributing to a particular decision and that evidence in itself cannot determine policy, particularly given the many different contexts in which decisions have to be taken. For example, at the very simplest, there are frequently situations in which relevant evidence is not available on the particular population sub-group of greatest interest to policy-makers.

Although the 'enlightenment' model does not explain in detail how research findings and ideas percolate into policy processes, it emphasizes that the relationship between evidence and policy is a social process and is consistent with the more explanatory theories of policy and decision processes provided by both political and management science. Pawson (2006: 175) quotes Mintzberg's (1976) description of decision-making as a 'recursive discontinuous process involving many different steps and a host of dynamic factors over a considerable period of time'. In turn, most policy decision-making processes are characterised as incremental, messy, open-ended, loosely structured and exploratory. They also involve resolving clashes of values and ideas articulated by different groups through the application of practical reasoning and argument. Lin (2003: 296) argues that policy is about 'exercising judgment in the face of uncertainty'. An obvious reason why policy decision-making involves a considerable amount of judgment is that it relates to the future which can only ever be partly known in advance. It is thus a creative process of imagination. As Pawson (2006: 171) points out, interventions will have diverse effects because of the different contexts in which they are tried out and future interventions are likely to differ in detail from anything so far seen and so will have effects that cannot be fully predicted. All of these insights are largely consistent with the 'enlightenment' model.

The final implication of the 'enlightenment' model that is especially relevant to those who wish to take action to increase the likelihood that evidence will be used for policy and management decision-making is that there are very many potential points of contact between those involved in producing evidence and those involved in decision-making as the findings and ideas from research filter into the policy environment. Weiss (1979) argued that the more interaction there was between whosoever the 'policy-makers' were in a particular situation and researchers, the more likely the evidence produced from research would be taken seriously by policy-makers. These insights have been seized on by those who wish to encourage the use of evidence to recommend a variety of different ways of building formal and informal connections and relationships in different ways between researchers and policy-makers (Hanney et al. 2003). The current emphasis is on encouraging and helping evidence producers to 'push' their findings and the 'users' to make more informed demands for better evidence, while at the same time encouraging more 'linkage and exchange' between the two (Lavis et al. 2003).

'Linkage and exchange' and the 'two communities' model

The focus on 'linkage and exchange' is based on the simple idea that researchers and policy-makers or managers represent 'two communities' with different values and interests, different ways of seeing the world and understanding how it works, and different goals and methods of working. This idea is inherently plausible. For example, there is no doubt that the two groups use different languages, have different career trajectories, encounter different institutional incentives and constraints, have different priorities and espouse different views about the significance of research. Table 7.2 summarises the main differences in stylised fashion.

This 'two communities' model focuses particular attention on the barriers that lie in the way of transferring research into policy in terms of the need for

Table 7.2 The 'two communities' model of researchers and policy makers (Buse et al. 2005 adapted)

	Researchers	Policy makers
Work	Discrete, planned research projects using explicit, scientific methods designed to produce unambiguous, generalisable results (knowledge focused); usually highly specialised in research areas and knowledge	Continuous, unplanned flow of tasks involving negotiation and compromise between interests and goals, assessment of practical feasibility of policies and advice on specific decisions (decision focused). Often required to work on a range of different issues simultaneously
Attitudes to research	Justified by its contribution to valid knowledge; research findings lead to need for further investigations	Only one of many inputs to their work; justified by its relevance and practical utility (e.g. in decision-making); some scepticism of findings versus their own experience
Accountability	To scientific peers primarily, but also to funders	To politicians primarily, but also the public, indirectly
Priorities	Expansion of research opportunities and influence of experts in the world	Maintaining a system of 'good governance' and satisfying politicians
Careers/rewards	Built largely on publication in peer reviewed scientific journals and peer recognition rather than practical impact	Built on successful management of complex political processes rather than use of research findings for policy
Training and knowledge base	High level of training, usually specialised within a single discipline; little knowledge about policy making	Often, though not always, generalists expected to be flexible; little or no scientific training
Organisational constraints	Relatively few (except resources); high level of discretion e.g. in choice of research focus	Embedded in large, inter-dependent bureaucracies and working within political limits, often to short timescales
Values/orientation	Place high value on independence of thought and action; belief in unbiased search for generalisable knowledge	Oriented to providing high quality advice, but attuned to a particular context and specific decisions

better translation, dissemination and communication of research findings. It also highlights the idea that there is a 'gap' between the two communities that must be spanned, for example, by people whose role is to act as 'brokers' or 'boundary spanners' managing difficulties in translation, and bringing the demand and supply of evidence into equilibrium.

Weiss's insights and the notion of 'two communities' have been used to develop a range of practical methods of trying to change the ways in which researchers and policy-makers interact before, during and after the undertaking of research in order to increase the odds of research being used more directly and immediately in the policy process than the 'enlightenment' model suggests is often the case. Table 7.3 summarises some of the most obvious ways of attempting to reduce the supposed 'gap' between research being undertaken and its findings being used for policy and management decision-making which would apply as much to systematic reviews as other forms of evidence synthesis. Note that it specifically mentions reviews as forms of research that

Table 7.3 Some practical steps commonly advocated to reduce the 'gap' between research and policy (Buse et al. 2005 adapted)

Steps to be taken by researchers	Steps to be taken by policy makers
Provide a range of different types of research report including newsletters, executive summaries, short policy papers, etc. all written in an accessible, jargon-free style, specific to the particular context and easily available (e.g. by hiring a scientific journalist to translate research reports into lay terms or training researchers in accessible writing styles suitable to different audiences). Include potentially actionable messages based on the findings even if specific recommendations are not appropriate	Set up formal communication channels and advisory mechanisms involving researchers and policy makers (and the public) to identify research priorities, researchable questions, develop research designs, and jointly plan the dissemination and use of findings
Put on conferences, seminars, briefings and practical workshops to disseminate research findings and educate policy makers about research	
Produce interim reports to ensure that findings are timely	
Include specific policy implications in research reports (though check that these are required and would be welcomed)	Ensure that all major policies and programmes are preceded by systematic reviews of relevant evidence and have evaluations built into their budgets and implementation plans rather than seeing evaluation as an optional extra

Identify 'knowledge champions', opinion leaders and innovators, and ensure that they understand the implications of research findings and can act as credible 'messengers' or intermediaries

Undertake systematic reviews of research findings on policy-relevant questions to enable policy makers to access information more easily

Publish the findings of all public programme evaluations and view evaluation as an opportunity for policy learning

Keep in close contact with potential policy makers throughout the research process, including in some cases involving policy staff directly in the review

Commission research and evaluation directly and consider having additional in-house research capacity

Design studies and reviews to maximise their policy relevance and utility (e.g. ensure that trials are of interventions feasible in a wide range of settings)

Establish intermediate institutions designed to review research and determine its policy and management implications (e.g. the National Institute for Health and Clinical Excellence in England and Wales which advises patients, health professionals and the NHS on current 'best practice' derived from robust evidence syntheses)

Use a range of research and synthesis methods, including 'action-research' (i.e. participative, practically-oriented, non-exploitative research which directly involves the subjects of research at all stages with a view to producing new knowledge that empowers people to improve their situation) and other innovative methods

Provide more opportunities for the public and civil society organisations to learn about the nature of research, to be able to ask questions of researchers and policy makers concerning the use of research and to participate more actively in the policy process from an informed position

Choose research topics that are important for future policy

Encourage the mass media to improve the quality of their reporting and interpretation of research findings and their policy implications through devoting more time and effort to media briefing

---

should have particular attraction for likely end users on the grounds that they make large bodies of evidence highly accessible.

The issue of how to present the findings of reviews to increase their accessibility to policy and management audiences was discussed in Chapter 6. While presentation is clearly important, good communication and dissemination of findings are almost never sufficient to get evidence taken notice of and have to be complemented by a number of other more 'active' strategies, since research is only ever one input to policy and management processes. Those strategies most specific to reviews are discussed below.

Making the review relevant

The principal ways in which a review can be made relevant to potential management and policy users relate to the selection of review objectives and questions, the range of evidence included and the choice of synthesis methods. Lavis et al. (2005) surveyed a range of senior decision-makers in the UK and Canada about their interest in, and likely use of, systematic reviews, and concluded that they wanted rigorous reviews that were potentially reproducible, using trustworthy, transparent methods, intelligible to a lay audience. These decision-makers generally assumed that researchers knew their business and did not want to have to second-guess them, rather they preferred to select reviewers whom they could trust, particularly when the synthesis methods depended on a considerable amount of judgment (e.g. realist synthesis). They simply wished to be assured that the reviews were of good quality. In addition, they asked for relevant, up-to-date answers to their questions in their context or population using whatever definition of 'evidence' helped answer their questions, including experiential knowledge. In other words, they placed a premium on the availability of locally relevant and useable knowledge.

Pawson et al. (2005) argue that time spent discussing, negotiating and refining the questions for reviews is essential to the production of useable reviews. Pawson (2006) argues that realist synthesis, in particular, tries to build theories which take into account the context of programme implementation as well as the conceptual world of the decision-makers. By contrast, Davies (1999) reminds researchers that sometimes what policy-makers need to know is not what they initially want to know and that some delicate persuasion may be necessary to help them clarify and revise their questions. As a result, it is worth spending time trying to find out what the decision-makers are trying to achieve and to identify their underlying theory of how this will be accomplished. At the same time, the review team needs to identify questions that are also answerable with the methods and evidence available.

As discussed in Chapter 2, the early stages of the review are also the opportunity to clarify whether the review is primarily designed to support a particular decision ('decision support' role) or whether it is designed to provide an overview of relevant knowledge ('knowledge support'). The latter is likely to provide more of a background function and is, by definition, less likely to be directly useable for decision-making in a specific context. This is because: 'Best problem solutions, if found at all, are appropriate or best to a time and place . . . The timeless universal solutions sought in some versions of scientific problem solving do not exist' (Lindblom 1990: 224). Choosing a 'decision support' role affects not only the methods of synthesis and range of evidence likely to be employed (e.g. there is more need to incorporate assumptions and valuations from policy-makers and stakeholders alongside research evidence in 'decision support' reviews), it also has implications for the working of the review team. For example, the range of skills required in a 'decision support' review is likely to be wider since the review team is more likely to be involved in activities that are directly linked to the decision-making process. Decision oriented reviews are also more likely to directly involve representatives of the end-users in the research team since they may well have access to information unavailable elsewhere.

In terms of the content of reviews, Lavis et al. (2005) highlighted the fact that senior policy-makers and managers wanted findings and conclusions of interventions to be expressed in terms of benefits, harms (or risks) and costs for the population as a whole and sub-groups, as well as wanting highlighted the degree of uncertainty associated with each of the estimates made. They argued that users of reviews did not necessarily require recommendations for action in all cases, but that this would depend what had been agreed in advance, and what the purpose of the review was (e.g. 'decision support' versus 'knowledge support').

Timeliness

Political scientists frequently refer to the idea that major policy change can occur only when a 'window of opportunity' opens in the policy process (Kingdon 1997). Such 'windows' are time-limited indicating that relevant research has to be available at the right time to contribute to policy decisions. It can be difficult to predict how and when 'windows of opportunity' will open, but it is a basic requirement that the research team understands from the outset how pressing the need for the review is and whether there is a deadline beyond which the findings will be far less useful. If timescales are short, but also uncertain, it may be advisable to consider producing an interim synthesis and draft set of conclusions before going on to complete the full review. Another, related approach is to undertake a rapid 'scoping' exercise and report it at an early stage (Davies 1999). Good liaison arrangements with potential decision-makers (who may have commissioned the review) should help the review team stay informed of any changes in an agreed timetable driven by external factors.

Building relationships

At the core of the 'linkage and exchange' approach to getting evidence used for decision-making are a range of ways of encouraging and planning interaction and liaison between researchers and policy-makers so that both are more likely to 'own' the conclusions. A variety of options has been proposed all of which are worth considering in different circumstances:

- development of 'brokerage' and liaison between researchers and policy-makers by recruiting specific staff whose task it is to link researchers and decision-makers by improving communication and mutual understanding;

- funding of programmes of synthesis rather than individual projects so that researchers and potential users become familiar with each other's ways of thinking and working;

- exchanges and secondments between research centres and policy agencies so that more researchers can gain decision-making experience and more decision-makers can develop a better knowledge of how research is undertaken, and its strengths and limitations;

- co-location of decision-makers and research analysts during projects, perhaps involving research which is jointly produced and disseminated;

- undertaking a 'stakeholder analysis' alongside the review process to identify in advance which organisations, interest groups and individuals are likely to be most influential in terms of whether the findings of the review are taken seriously.

While 'brokerage', exchanges, co-location and co-production of reviews can all contribute to building relationships between review teams and decision-makers, thereby increasing the odds of use of the findings, they all depend on there being regular face-to-face meetings between the two to discuss the direction, content, emerging findings, presentation and potential applicability of reviews. To make the most of these meetings, there needs to be a reasonably high degree of trust and openness in both directions. One role for such meetings is for the review team to be able to test out its conclusions and any recommendations (if these were asked for) with the relevant decision-makers in terms of whether they are feasible and expressed in a way that can be acted upon in the relevant context (Pawson et al. 2005: 24). Another role is for potential decision-makers to explain where they think they have reached in the process of policy development, what is 'given' and what is potentially alterable in light of evidence. Another function of meetings is to enable the review team to gain an informal understanding of the values driving the policy process and the relative weights key stakeholders attribute to particular outcomes or effects of policy.

Beyond the 'two communities' model

The 'two communities' model and the related focus on 'linkage and exchange' have been extremely helpful in sensitising researchers and policy-makers to the practical barriers that can limit the use of research findings to influence policy and management decisions. The model has helped in developing practical responses that serve to narrow the 'gap' between the different worlds of research, policy and management by improving the flow of credible knowledge between groups of people who would otherwise have difficulty interacting and communicating. The 'linkage and exchange' movement exemplified by the work of the Canadian Health Services Research Foundation (www.chsrf.ca) represents perhaps the most sophisticated response to date to the frustrations inherent in the relationship between research, policy and management. The approach has the great strength of seeing policy and management not as a series of discrete steps that includes a specific, easily identifiable decision point (which researchers can try to affect), but rather as a continuous process involving a range of groups, taking place within a particular set of institutional relationships. CHSRF, for example, recognises in its work that there will be differences of view between different policy agencies and individuals involved in the policy process, encouraging researchers to be careful to identify different target groups for their messages and to use appropriate strategies to reach each group. Various forms of innovative 'linkage and exchange' are being tested experimentally with encouraging results in Canada (Denis and Lomas 2003).

However, seen from the perspective of policy science, 'linkage and exchange' methods still tend to see the underlying problem fundamentally in terms of the separation between two distinct worlds with different values, facing different incentives and working in different ways. By contrast, policy scientists have radically challenged the accuracy and thus usefulness of the concept of 'two communities':

> This construction has endured for three decades because it resonates with the experience of many researchers and policy-makers. But what if the two communities phenomenon was not the real driver of the nexus between research and policy? What if it was a reasonable description of the experience of researchers and policy-makers, but a poor explanation for why there are problems in the research–policy relationship? What if it has become a self-fulfilling prophecy rather than a fruitful basis for renewed effort?
>
> (Gibson 2003: 19)

Gibson sensitises us, instead, to the existence of conflicts among researchers, and also among policy-makers and managers, as well as the commonalities and alliances between sub-groups of researchers and decision-makers. Anyone who has ever attended an academic conference from outside academia will have been struck by the extent of debate, dispute and controversy between rival groups of researchers and theorists. Likewise, researchers who hold particular positions in academic debates are more or less likely to be regarded sympathetically by policy-makers and managers who either do or do not share the same underlying assumptions. For example, both researchers and policy-makers will differ in the emphasis they give in their explanations of human behaviour to individual choice (e.g. in terms of its contribution to differences in health between individuals and social groups over the life course). This, in turn, will affect the kinds of research they undertake or commission, as well as the findings and policy solutions that they find immediately convincing and those which they will respond to sceptically. In turn, this will affect their perception of who is 'in tune' with their way of thinking and who is not. In the case of a policy-maker with some influence over the funding of research, this may translate into a bias in favour of supporting certain kinds of inquiry or research undertaken from a particular disciplinary or theoretical perspective. In the case of a researcher with a longstanding interest in a particular issue (e.g. the factors shaping health differences over the life course), this may translate into seeking to cultivate politicians, officials and managers who share the same underlying beliefs about the importance of the early years of life in order to build alliances to develop policy and research.

From this perspective, the starting point for the analysis of the relation-ship between 'research' and 'policy' is a general understanding of the policy process rather than a specific focus on the 'two communities' assumed to be salient. There are a number of different ways of thinking about the public policy process each of which suggests different constructions of the research–policy/management relationship, and each of which has some empirical sup-port. Two of them are described here. The first understands the policy process in terms of interactions between participants in policy networks and policy communities and the second, develops this idea and sees the process in terms of the interaction of advocacy coalition. Both have the merit of seeing researchers as political actors within the policy process, building support for their policy proposals and research interests rather than as a separate, homo-geneous group outside the process trying to exert their influence. This avoids the potentially damaging assumption made by many researchers that they can see the policy issues from a uniquely objective position by virtue of their research accomplishments and that they should, therefore, be deferred to.

Policy networks and policy communities

These approaches to understanding how decisions are taken focus attention on the patterns of formal and informal relationships that shape ideas and proposals for action, as well as decisions. For example, whether a policy issue ever reaches the policy agenda of a government agency (i.e. comes to be regarded as a priority for analysis and attention) is seen from this perspective as the result of the interactions between individuals and groups, including researchers of various types, organised in differing degrees of formality around specific policy areas and issues. In general, analysts tend to use the term policy community to refer to relatively stable, restricted and formal constellations of organisations and actors that cohere around a particular field of policy (e.g. treatment of people with schizophrenia). The 'policy community' thus mainly comprises policy 'insiders' (i.e. participants who have an established position relatively close to government). The term policy network tends to indicate a much looser, less stable, less restricted set of individuals and interest groups focusing on a policy area. Therefore, the 'policy network' is likely to include more 'outsider' groups as well as more established organisations closer to government. In reality, there is a continuum between policy communities and policy networks in terms of ease of entry and the degree of formality of relationships between groups.

The nature of the policy network or community around an issue (e.g. tight versus loose; highly integrated versus loosely bound together; inward looking versus open to new ideas) will shape the way that researchers participate and the way that evidence from research is regarded and taken into account. Clearly, in a tightly knit, stable community, the key step for a researcher is to become regarded as a legitimate 'insider' in order to have a chance of being listened to. In a more fluid network, the key skill from the point of view of a researcher who wishes to exert influence is to be able to recognise new participants in the network at an early stage, get to know their interests and views, and develop some form of relationship with them. The looser the network, the more divergent are the views represented and the wider the range of different types of research that are likely to be seen as legitimate and useable by those advocating different policy solutions (Nutley and Webb 2000).

Whatever the situation, this broad perspective sees all those involved in the network or community as potential 'policy-makers' rather than starting with a strong prior assumption that there are separate groups of 'researchers' and 'policy-makers'. The identity of the 'policy-makers' or 'policy influentials' is an empirical issue rather than a 'given' associated with those who occupy official positions. It only becomes apparent through studying the policy process who is influential and why.

The advocacy coalition framework (ACF)

The ACF represents a development of policy network and policy community theories based on considerable research in the USA. Under this approach, each policy field is seen as comprising a large number of actors (at first sight, a network or community) which, on further investigation, can be seen as organised into a smaller number of distinct, relatively stable 'advocacy coalitions' in conflict with one another (Sabatier and Jenkins-Smith 1993). Each coalition competes for the ear of government in this model. Each is distinguished empirically by having a distinct set of norms, beliefs and resources. Crucially, for the current discussion, each 'coalition' (as the name suggests) is likely to comprise a diverse range of politicians, civil servants, members of civil society organisations, researchers, journalists and others. Advocacy coalitions are thus defined by their shared ideas rather than by the work their members do or by the roles their members fulfil in decision-making institutions or by their formal organisational memberships. Within such coalitions there is consensus about fundamental policy goals and positions, though there may be more debate about the detail of the means to achieve these goals. The 'core' beliefs of advocacy coalitions change relatively infrequently and in response to major changes in the environment outside the specific policy field. 'Normal' policy change is identified as the result of learning, debate and interaction between advocacy coalitions within the policy system. Each advocacy coalition interprets and uses research findings to advance its distinct policy goals in different ways.

From the point of view of the role of researchers and research in policy and management decisions, one particularly important facet of the ACF relates to the existence of so-called 'policy brokers'. Analysis of case studies of policy change identifies special actors who are concerned to find acceptable, feasible compromises between the positions adopted by the different advocacy coalitions at work in a particular field of policy. The identity of these 'brokers' becomes apparent only after the event, but, most obviously, they include bodies set up specifically to generate agreement such as commissions of inquiry or consensus development conferences. Such bodies and related processes offer researchers opportunities to get their research taken seriously. However, much 'brokerage' is undertaken informally and is not the product of any conscious decision-making on the part of government or policy officials.

Implications for research and policy

Theories of the policy process that abandon the 'two communities' perspective significantly alter the focus of attention for those wishing to increase the impact of research on policy and management decisions. Gibson (2003) identifies four implications of these theories. First, researchers who wish to influence policy must analyse the policy area politically to identify the advocacy coalitions and policy communities, and their core values and beliefs about the nature of the policy problem, its causes and potential solutions (technical analysis of the content of policy change is not enough). Second, researchers must be engaged directly with advocacy coalitions or policy communities if they wish to have influence rather than focusing exclusively on managing the boundary and reducing the 'gap' between two worlds of research and policy activities. Third, research evidence owes its influence in the policy process to its ability to be turned into arguments and advocacy by actors and often self-appointed 'brokers' in the policy process rather than its ability to reveal an uncontested 'truth'. And finally a strategy to enhance the role of research in policy is as much about influencing values and beliefs, and producing good arguments as it is about improving the knowledge base and its transmission.

Drawbacks of pursuing the 'use' of evidence

If Gibson's analysis is correct, it is challenging, particularly for researchers. It means getting much more closely involved in the policy process and in developing convincing arguments rather relying on the evidence 'speaking for itself' than many researchers are either temperamentally or ethically pre-pared to do. Researchers have to decide whether they wish to adopt an 'insider' (e.g. seeking to become an accepted and trusted adviser to govern-ment or other policy actors) or 'outsider' (e.g. achieving prominence as a fear-less critic or supporter of particular policy positions operating in a public manner) strategy to achieve influence. It exposes researchers to the risk that they will have to over-simplify their findings and the implications of their research in order to guarantee an audience unwilling to engage with the com-plexity and ambiguity of the evidence. As Pawson (2006: 176) uncomfortably reminds us, the evidence from reviews is like all evidence, 'partial, provisional and conditional' – hardly the stuff to get the media and politicians on the edge of their seats. Instead, researchers may find themselves under pressure to identify 'best buys' with a high degree of certainty. The final drawback for researchers of pursuing the 'use' of evidence is more subtle: it reinforces the false notion that more evidence in and of itself will reduce the inherent uncertainty of policy and management decisions, and reduce the need for judgements about what should be done as opposed to what appears to be known from the past.

Conclusions

Research is only one among a wide variety of influences on policy and man-agement processes. Yet, there is no doubt that the policy-making process is influenced by research: research can help define a phenomenon as a policy problem potentially worthy of attention and research provides 'enlighten-ment' with many ideas affecting policy-makers and managers indirectly and over long periods of time. This is facilitated by the links between policy-makers and researchers, the role of the media, timing and how the research is com-municated. There are also many impediments to research being acted upon, including political and ideological factors, policy uncertainty, uncertainty about scientific findings, the perceived utility of research and how easy it is to communicate. There is considerable enthusiasm at present for using a variety of brokerage and knowledge exchange mechanisms to improve the productivity of the relationship between researchers and policy-makers viewed as distinct communities.

However, the idea that researchers and policy-makers comprise two culturally distinct 'communities' is potentially misleading. Neither group is homogeneous and there are areas of common ground shared by some researchers and some policy-makers. Subsets of researchers and policy-makers participate together in competing 'advocacy coalitions' or 'policy networks' around issues. This perspective suggests that research enters policy as much through influencing political argument as through the transmission of knowledge. This indicates that recent efforts to use techniques of 'linkage' and 'exchange' to bridge the supposed 'gap' between research and policy are unlikely to succeed as much as their proponents would like.

8   Approaches and assessment: choosing different methods and considering quality

Part 1 of this book looked at the reasons for undertaking reviews and synthesis of evidence. It outlined different types of review and the stages of a review for policy and management. Part 2 set out the main approaches to synthesis relevant to reviews of diverse evidence. This chapter aims to bring these two parts together by discussing how different methods and combinations of methods of synthesis may be relevant to different review questions and bodies of evidence, and thus how reviews as a whole may be designed and planned. The chapter concludes by discussing the quality of reviews of complex bodies of evidence for policy and management. Having chosen the specific approaches to synthesis in Part 2 and implemented the advice in Parts 1 and 2, how can one tell that a review is likely to be of good quality before it is accomplished or after completion?

Choosing and combining approaches to synthesis within reviews

The chapters in Part 2 described and assessed the relevance, strengths and limitations of a range of methods for synthesis which could be used in reviews of complex bodies of evidence for policy- and decision-making. It was noted in Part 1 that the kinds of question asked by policy and/or management decision-makers were likely to require the inclusion of a wide range of evidence (qualitative and quantitative, research and non-research). As a result, reviews for policy- and decision-making are likely to employ more than one synthesis method, reflecting the different types of evidence identified as relevant to the range of questions asked. This raises two questions: which approaches to synthesis should be used for which purposes and in which circumstances; and which combinations are most effective for which purposes and in which circumstances? The latter question raises some of the same issues encountered in the design of mixed method primary research studies in the social sciences;

that is, individual studies that include both qualitative and quantitative elements of data collection and analysis. In primary applied research in the social sciences, such as in the health field, the desire of researchers, funders and policy-makers to answer a wider range of questions in a single study has led to considerable use of mixed methods (O'Cathain and Thomas 2006). For example, a common impetus towards mixed methods studies is the desire to know not only whether a specific intervention 'works' (its effectiveness), but also how it works, where it works best and why, and how most effectively to develop and transfer the intervention elsewhere. Clearly qualitative research is extremely helpful in understanding how an intervention produces its effects, to what extent this may be due to unique versus more general circumstances and what implications this has for implementing the intervention in other settings.

Just as in primary research where researchers should provide an explicit rationale for their choice of methods of data collection, so too reviewers need to justify the synthesis method or methods they choose, and work out how they are going to use these approaches to best advantage. The evidence represents the raw material that the review team has to work with and is a major influence on the possible synthesis methods. Given the range of types of evidence that can be required for policy- and decision-making, it is possible that any of the methods of synthesis described in Part 2 or combinations of methods will be appropriate, depending on the specific requirements of a review. It may not be possible at the outset of the review process to define the synthesis methods exactly (e.g. the precise nature of the evidence in the field may be largely unknown at the start), but it should become clearer once the review questions are defined, and the scope of the review and nature of the relevant evidence have been identified which methods of synthesis in what sequence are likely to be most fruitful.

As discussed in Chapter 1, some researchers take the view that qualitative and quantitative research methods cannot be 'mixed' in either primary research or systematic reviews, on the grounds that they are based on different philosophical positions on the nature of social reality and how knowledge about the social world can be attained (i.e. what is knowable). In contrast, this book is based on a 'subtle realist' perspective (Hammersley 1992) that allows the use of both qualitative and quantitative methods and data in primary studies, and by extension, in reviews and synthesis. From this perspective, different synthesis methods, if well used, can generate insights and ideas that cannot be derived from single approaches. Even so, care has to be taken when planning to use combinations of different methods in reviews or primary studies. There are a number of important questions to be answered at the design stage, including:

• Which method(s) are necessary in this review and why?

- How do the methods relate to the questions posed?
- What specifically will be gained by using this particular method or combination of methods?
- How will the different methods be sequenced or will they be undertaken simultaneously?
- Who will do the analyses using the different approaches – the same members of the team or different members for each approach?
- When and how will the findings from different synthesis methods be used?
- Will different methods be given more or less priority in the final analysis?
- Is the intention to try to integrate the findings or to contrast them?
- What analytic and interpretive strategy will be used if different methods produce different 'answers' to the same question(s)?

These questions draw attention to the fact that there are a number of different ways in which quantitative, interpretive and 'mixed' (e.g. narrative) approaches to synthesis can be used in a single review, just as they might be used in primary studies, depending on the underlying aim (e.g. overview of research for knowledge support versus contribution to a 'verdict' as part of decision-making), specific questions to be tackled, the nature and balance of the evidence available (e.g. whether most of the evidence is derived from qualitative or quantitative or mixed method research) and the stage that policy development has reached. For instance, quantitative syntheses of effectiveness or cost-effectiveness (e.g. some form of meta-analysis) might be more relevant if there was genuine uncertainty as to which among a range of interventions should be implemented, whereas an interpretive synthesis (e.g. meta-ethnography) might be more useful at a later stage to explain the barriers and limitations to a particular type of intervention, as a way of informing the design of an intervention already identified as the most cost-effective from prior research and how it should be implemented. Where decision-makers are at an early stage in trying to devise an entirely new intervention, a realist review designed to help develop the 'theory' underlying the intervention (i.e. a plausible account of how the intervention might be expected to work) might be most appropriate.

Table 8.1 attempts to provide some guidance as to which approaches and combinations of approaches to synthesis are likely to be most suitable for different sorts of review aims, questions and evidence. Both 'mixed' synthesis approaches (e.g. narrative synthesis, realist synthesis etc, described in Chapter 5) and Bayesian approaches (described in Chapter 3) are likely to be appropriate for reviews with more of a decision support function because they can more easily encompass research and non-research evidence. Interpretive (Chapter 4) and some of the other quantitative (e.g. case survey,

Table 8.1 Choosing a suitable approach to synthesis given the aim, questions and evidence of the review (Mays et al. 2005 adapted)

Review aim and/or policy/ management question	Relevant types of evidence (if available)	Likely approach(es) to synthesis	Strengths of the approach	Limits to the approach
'Knowledge support'	All types, but mostly research-based because of focus on what the research evidence says	All bar decision analysis, etc.	Generalisability	Does not directly help with a specific decision in a particular context
'Decision support'	All types, including research and non-research (i.e. need to know evidence, values and preferences of stakeholders and decision makers)	Bayesian meta-analysis, decision analysis, modelling and simulation of various types and possibly narrative synthesis	Focuses on the specifics of a particular decision in a particular context	Has to be modified to be relevant to another context; utility depends on its being used by decision-makers; not generalisable
Is this a problem?	All types including research and non-research (e.g. qualitative and quantitative research, public and stakeholder views, opinion polls, focus groups)	Narrative synthesis or, for qualitative studies, meta-ethnography	Narrative synthesis is flexible, relatively easy to understand and applicable to a range of situations and sources of evidence; meta-ethnography has principally been used for qualitative synthesis	Have to work hard to make sure methods and judgments are explicit, free of bias and replicable; defining something as a 'problem' is value-laden
How big is the problem? Which groups does it affect?	Quantitative research and routine data analysis. Qualitative data on subjective impact	Quantitative synthesis plus meta-ethnography of qualitative studies		Meta-ethnography is labour intensive, requires considerable qualitative research experience
Is it changing over time?	Quantitative research and routine data analysis	Quantitative synthesis		

What can be done about it (what may work)? How much is responding likely to cost in general?	Mostly quantitative research on effectiveness and cost-effectiveness	Meta-analysis of intervention studies	Meta-analysis well developed for effectiveness and reasonably well developed for cost-effectiveness data	
How do the seemingly effective policies or interventions work?	Mostly qualitative research from interviews and observation on users' and providers' experiences	Various forms of interpretive synthesis (e.g. qualitative cross-case analysis or meta-ethnography), but also realist synthesis	Rich picture of how policies or interventions work in practice as opposed to preconceptions of their architects	Qualitative studies may not have been undertaken in relevant settings so findings may be hard to apply
What works, for whom, in which circumstances? What factors may moderate the impact of this policy?	Wide range of research and non-research data	Realist synthesis; narrative synthesis; case survey	Helps with understanding mechanisms underlying interventions (i.e. how they work)	Will not necessarily produce specific answers to particular decision needs
Will intervention/policy x work here with what cost and benefit consequences?	Cost-effectiveness data from research; modelling related to specific circumstances including non-research data	Bayesian meta-analysis and cost-effectiveness modelling; decision analysis	Makes research evidence relevant to specific circumstances of a particular decision	Dependent on validity of expert opinion where research is lacking and on specific value trade-offs of decision makers; decision makers may be reluctant to follow 'verdict' of the analysis; Bayesian meta-analysis can be hard to explain

(continued overleaf)

Table 8.1 (continued)

Review aim and/or policy/ management question	Relevant types of evidence (if available)	Likely approach(es) to synthesis	Strengths of the approach	Limits to the approach
How acceptable will intervention/policy x be? Will it be implemented successfully? What will the reaction be here?	Largely qualitative research and non-research data (e.g. focus groups, opinion polls, stakeholder analysis)	Interpretive synthesis (e.g. meta-ethnography, qualitative cross-case analysis etc.)	Essential information for policy makers and managers even though tricky to interpret	'Softness' and/or transitory nature of opinions and views

Chapter 3) approaches described in this book were primarily designed for synthesis of research and so are more suited to the knowledge support role. In general, the various mixed methods discussed in Chapter 5 appear to offer the most flexibility to support both knowledge and decision-support functions.

A review may comprise a combination of approaches to synthesis as suggested in Chapter 5 and in Table 8.1, primarily so that a wide enough range of evidence can be brought to bear on a policy or management issue to answer the range of questions that may need attention (though there are other purposes, see below). The different approaches can also be sequenced in a number of ways. For example, a review of largely qualitative evidence might start with a thematic synthesis, but the richness of the evidence might lead the review team to consider undertaking a more ambitious meta-ethnography to develop a 'line of argument' synthesis to arrive at some higher-order interpretation which ties together the entire body of evidence available. In another review, a quantitative synthesis (e.g. using content analysis) or a narrative synthesis might generate additional questions that could be pursued by either an interpretive synthesis (e.g. to look at how a particular type of intervention is supposed to work) or a data-pooling method such as Bayesian meta-analysis (e.g. to look in more detail at its impact on particular sub-groups).

In principle, the main ways in which the different approaches to synthesis could be used in a single review are as follows:

1   to help answer different questions in the same review (and the more questions there are, for example, if they are both process and outcome related, the more different approaches are likely to be relevant);
2   to broaden the scope and depth of a review by allowing a wider range of evidence to be brought to bear on the same question(s);
3   to compare the findings from different methods of synthesis (e.g. it may be that the qualitative evidence is more focused on users' views of a service and the quantitative evidence is more focused on professionals' views and user outcomes, and these different perspectives need to brought together by using both interpretive and quantitative approaches to synthesis);
4   where an interpretive synthesis identifies new questions which may be answered through a quantitative synthesis or informs the design of the ensuing quantitative synthesis;
5   where quantitative synthesis helps establish the generalisability of insights derived from a previous interpretive synthesis;
6   when an interpretive synthesis provides an explanation of the findings from a quantitative synthesis (e.g. by providing an interpretation of variations in outcomes between RCTs included in a meta-analysis).

These uses have considerable similarities with the ways in which qualitative and quantitative methods are combined in primary social science research. In their discussion of the use of mixed methods in primary research, O'Cathain and Thomas (2006) identify three distinctly different purposes underpinning the use of mixed methods, which are equally applicable to combining different methods for synthesis in reviews.

First they suggest that the purpose of mixed methods can be 'complementarity' or 'extension'. This is the purpose behind many reviews that include both qualitative and quantitative evidence and focuses on getting 'more' of a picture of a phenomenon by looking at it from a number of different perspectives (Barbour 1999). The basic idea behind this justification for the use of interpretive and quantitative research and non-research evidence is that the whole can equate to more than simply the sum of the parts if the different sources are used creatively. The EPPI Centre approach discussed at the end of Chapter 5 is clearly based on the notion of 'complementarity' in that it explicitly includes a combination of approaches to synthesis within a single review. The EPPI Centre has undertaken a series of systematic reviews to identify the barriers to, and facilitators of, young people's mental health, physical activity, smoking and healthy eating, respectively. Each review attempts to integrate three different approaches to synthesis (Harden et al. 2004):

1   a quantitative synthesis of studies of effectiveness of health-promoting interventions using statistical meta-analysis (pooling data from different, comparable studies and calculating overall effect sizes of interventions), where appropriate;

2   an interpretive synthesis of studies of people's perceptions and experiences in which original studies are interrogated, re-analysed and combined to produce an overarching thematic analysis or 'theory' as to which kinds of interventions might work to promote the health of different kinds of people. The framework for the thematic analysis is shaped by the objectives of the review (i.e. to identify barriers and facilitating factors relevant to different health-related behaviours);

3   a final integrating synthesis which uses the results of the interpretive synthesis to interpret, add context to and refine the conclusions of the quantitative synthesis. This can involve further meta-analyses to test hypotheses about factors influencing the effectiveness of interventions. In the series of reviews looking at what influences different health-related behaviours and what can be done to alter these influences, the third synthesis attempted to answer the following question: to what extent do the interventions whose effectiveness was assessed in the first synthesis address the barriers identified by

young people and to what extent do they build upon the facilitators identified by young people as likely to improve mental health, physical activity, healthy eating and smoking in the second synthesis? In other words, the aim was to identify from among the effective interventions those most likely to work consistently with young people given their views and experiences of obstacles and enablers of healthy living.

The principles behind this combined approach are to preserve the distinctive contribution of each of the main types of evidence while also providing a way for each to help interpret the other so that a more comprehensive and useful answer to the review's main question can be provided. In the example above, this process enabled the review team to identify which subgroup of properly evaluated interventions was both effective and acceptable to young people and, therefore, most likely to produce sustained behavioural change.

The second purpose behind mixing methods identified by O'Cathain and Thomas (2006) is what they call 'development' – this is where methods are combined to enable one approach to assist another; for instance, where an interpretive approach is used to refine the question to be answered by a subsequent quantitative synthesis, or to contribute to the prior distribution in a Bayesian meta-analysis, or to identify a typology of interventions to be assessed later in terms of their cost-effectiveness. This purpose is associated particularly with the sequential use of different methods of synthesis in the same review.

O'Cathain and Thomas (2006) use the term 'crystallisation' in preference to 'triangulation' to refer to the third purpose of mixing methods. This is defined as a process of comparing different studies to explore the extent and nature of either convergence (with a focus on confirmation), divergence (e.g. identifying and studying 'deviant case' studies) or contradiction (apparent or real) between their findings and conclusions. With this purpose in mind, an interpretive synthesis could be used to shed light on the possible causes of heterogeneity between studies in a quantitative meta-analysis. The idea is to refine the overall explanation of the findings of all the different approaches to synthesis so that it can accommodate all or most of the evidence.

'Triangulation' is frequently used as a justification for using a mix of methods in primary research and also in reviews, but the term is used in social science in so many different ways that it has become denuded of meaning. Its origins lie in navigation where two observations of landmarks are used to plot a third location. Erzberger and Kelle (2003) argue persuasively that it is a highly problematic concept when applied to the social sciences. In its most common social science usage, it refers to comparing the findings from different methods or sources (in this case approaches to synthesis) to seek agreement as a form of 'validation' of one method by another. Unfortunately, it is not self-evident why different methods should produce the same answer, or, indeed, necessarily be capable of focusing on the same phenomena (e.g. it is simply not possible for an interpretive synthesis to generate frequency counts that can be compared with those from a quantitative synthesis). 'Triangulation' risks focusing the analyst excessively on similarities between sources and methods, since it assumes that the addition of a source or method is designed to confirm an existing interpretation. If there are differences between sources or methods, the 'triangulator' has no easy way of deciding which source or method is the 'correct' one. It seems wiser to admit the possibility from the outset that comparisons of findings derived from different sources using different methods of synthesis may converge, diverge or even contradict one another, and to be clear how these different results will be handled.

Combining different methods of synthesis and different bodies of evidence requires that the members of the research or review team are willing to respect the contribution of different forms of knowledge to the overall project and have agreed in advance, as far as possible, how the different perspectives should be handled. Unresolved tensions can arise within teams in the absence of a plan for handling the implications of different forms of synthesis. Riley et al. (2005) describe the dilemmas faced by the qualitative researchers involved in a mixed method primary research study when their insights into the way a community health intervention was being delivered in practice threatened the design assumptions of the effectiveness trial. No consideration had been given in advance to the possibility that the qualitative study conducted alongside the trial could have significant implications for the integrity of the trial itself to the extent of questioning the basis of the trial and indicating that it should be redesigned.

Assessing the quality of reviews of qualitative and quantitative evidence

As has been apparent in the preceding parts of this book, systematic reviews combining qualitative and quantitative evidence are still relatively uncommon and are at a relatively early stage of development. As a result, it is not possible or sensible to provide definitive quality criteria for them. Given the likelihood that more than one approach to synthesis will commonly be used in these sorts of review since they tend to cover a range of evidence, it may never be straightforward to provide overarching quality criteria that can be applied routinely to all parts of such reviews. For one thing, the reviews are likely to vary very considerably in aim, questions, data and synthesis methods.

Yet the users of the reviews need to know to what extent they can rely on their findings and conclusions; funders need to know if the work they paid for has been well done; and other researchers who may be basing their new primary research on reviews need some basis for trusting that the reviews are a fair summary of what is already known.

There are two distinct, but not mutually exclusive, ways of approaching the assessment of systematic reviews that attempt to draw on diverse evidence: use of criteria or indicators that are applicable to the review as a whole; and use of criteria or indicators that are applicable to each of the specific synthesis methods employed in the review. No formally developed criteria of quality exist for reviews of diverse evidence as a whole, though criteria of quality for mixed method primary research may be worth consideration (e.g. the framework developed by Caracelli and Riggin,1994, to assess the quality of mixed method evaluation). In relation to the different approaches to synthesis used within the wider review, quality criteria relevant to the specific types of study synthesized by each method will be highly relevant. Each method of synthesis can be assessed in a way appropriate to its quantitative or qualitative research tradition. Thus a meta-ethnography could be assessed in the same way as a primary ethnographic study, or using a modification of the criteria applicable to qualitative research in general such as those developed by Spencer et al. (2003) and summarised in Mays and Pope (2006: 94–8). Likewise, there are quality assessment frameworks for meta-analysis and other quantitative methods for reviewing (Khan et al. 2001).

However, knowing that each of the component syntheses is of good quality still does not indicate whether the review as a whole has been well done or whether the other stages of the review are appropriate. For example, there may be faults in the way that the search for evidence was specified and accomplished, even if the ensuing syntheses were well done.

Questions to ask of a review for policy and management

Below is a series of questions relating to the main activities and stages of a systematic review of qualitative and quantitative evidence which could be used to assess the protocol before starting the review or to appraise the finished product:

1 Is the aim of the review clear (i.e. is the review clearly located on the continuum between pure 'knowledge support' (e.g. enlightenment, insight, effectiveness, or background orientation) on the one hand and exclusively 'decision support' (going beyond synthesizing the research evidence to offer, assess and recommend policy options in a specific decision context) on the other)?

2 Are the review questions, or objectives, if specific questions are not appropriate, relevant to the concerns of the relevant policy-makers

and managers in the particular setting; specifically, is there evidence that potential users of the review (these could be policy-makers, managers or patients, depending on the circumstances) were involved in specifying and/or developing the questions with the review team?

3 Do the reviewers show that they understand the importance of context for the interpretation and applicability of the evidence synthesized and that they understand the specific context in which the review's conclusions are intended to be used?

4 Are the methods explicitly and comprehensibly described so that others could follow them, if required (though not necessarily to produce the same results)?

5 Is each step in the review and adaptation of the protocol clearly justified? At the outset it may be difficult to set down all the methods and activities precisely since it is appropriate for complex reviews to evolve as they are undertaken (see Chapter 2), but after the review, it is important to be able to provide a thorough account of how the methods developed, and how key judgements and decisions were made and why. In particular, are there signs of informed judgement rather than the mechanical application of pre-set rules? Where judgements are made on the basis of the evidence, is the reasoning underpinning the judgements made clear so that it can be discussed, and challenged and revised, if found wanting?

6 In relation to the stages and elements of the review:
   (a) Are the searches comprehensive or purposively sampled, and up to date, bearing in mind the resources available and the likely yield from extending them?

   (b) Is there an appropriate 'fit' between the questions posed and the type(s) and sources of evidence assembled for the review; i.e. does the review include a sufficiently wide and relevant scope of evidence?

   (c) Are individual studies and other sources of evidence critically appraised for relevance and quality, either in advance or in use during the review process?

   (d) If exclusion and inclusion criteria are used, are these appropriate?

   (e) Is the choice of synthesis methods appropriate and, if more than one, does each clearly contribute to the conclusions (e.g. do the combined methods add to the ability to answer the review's questions, for example by contributing to 'crystallisation')?

(f)   If non-research evidence is included (e.g. decision-makers' values and views on issues for which there is no relevant research) is this carried out scientifically (e.g. are formal methods of deliberative process and data collection such as Delphi, nominal groups, formal community consultations and focus groups used) and is the quality of the non-research evidence also assessed (Lomas et al. 2005)?

(g)   How is the non-research evidence integrated into the overall analyses?

7   Is there evidence that the different types of knowledge are combined effectively to answer the key questions, or are different sources synthesized separately with little sign of an attempt at 'integration'; i.e. does the review generate new knowledge and insights as against simply assembling the existing knowledge; does the review fully exploit the potential breadth and variety of evidence and methods of synthesis available; is there any sign that the findings from one source or approach to synthesis are used to inform the analysis or interpretation of another source or approach (e.g. Thomas et al., 2004, from the EPPI Centre report how sub-groups identified in an interpretive review helped to explain the heterogeneity of findings from a parallel quantitative synthesis)?

8   If more than one approach to synthesis is included are they sequenced or carried out simultaneously to maximise the odds of answering the questions posed (e.g. are there signs of a deliberate strategy to precede a by b, or b by a, or to alternate the two – a b a or b a b, O'Cathain and Thomas 2006)?

9   If more than one approach to synthesis is included, how is the resultant analysis handled; i.e. is there an expectation that each approach will corroborate the other or is there an expectation of divergence between the different approaches; how are divergences and even contradictions handled if they arise (e.g. are explanations offered for divergences between the different methods and sources or are divergences seen as indicating a lack of validity on the part of one or another source and is this an appropriate conclusion to reach)?

10   Are the overall conclusions and/or explanation consistent with all the evidence from all the syntheses?

11   Is the review reported in a brief, lucid, non-technical way for the relevant policy and management audiences; if there are technical parts of the report, are these 'translated' for a non-researcher audience?

12 If guidance and/or recommendations are included, are they action-able (e.g. are they sufficiently specific to be capable of feasibility assessment)?

13 Does the review team include the range of disciplines, skills, subject area knowledge and experience of policy or management needed successfully to answer the questions posed with the evidence avail-able (e.g. if the review is predominantly for 'decision support' does the team include relevant decision-makers as advisers)?

These 13 questions are suggestions only, designed to help reviewers and potential users think about important aspects of the quality of reviews which encompass qualitative and quantitative evidence of various types. There may be other specific questions that become salient in relation to specific reviews. They are a start in a relatively untried process.

Conclusion: the case for synthesis

This book has outlined a range of different ways of synthesizing diverse sources of evidence to inform policy- and decision-making. The focus of the examples used to illustrate how this might be achieved have largely been derived from health care, but the broader principles and methods are likely to be applicable in wider social policy fields. The premise of the book has been that the kinds of questions asked by policy-makers, managers and practitioners are often complex, and the answers are likely to be found in a variety of sources of evidence. However this evidence does not come neatly packaged; it has to be collected, arranged and interpreted.

Within social science, education and health research, methods for under-taking reviews of evidence have been developed to bring together research evidence. The development of 'second generation' literature reviews and systematic reviews of effectiveness has begun to establish cumulative know-ledge or an evidence base in a number of areas. The methods available for reviewing have also improved, becoming more systematic and rigorous. But these reviews have often been confined to research evidence. Policy- and decision-makers may need to draw on evidence in the widest sense – different kinds of research findings, views of stakeholders and of expert panels and publics. Many of these reviews have also typically been focused on a single type of research evidence – the results of RCTs or other experimental methods or the qualitative literature on a particular topic and here again these may not always be appropriate to the needs of policy- and decision-makers.

This book has argued that synthesis offers a way of combining and inte-grating evidence; in particular, it has the potential to make a whole that is greater than the sum of the parts. Synthesis can also help with the process of 'getting evidence into practice and policy' – whether by providing an overview of the evidence as knowledge support, or in some instances by playing a more direct part through the use of the decision analysis. However, many of the methods for synthesis are evolving too. The majority were devised to synthesize either qualitative or quantitative research, and/or for analysing primary data. Few methods have been tested on the wide range of types of evidence which might be of interest to policy-makers and managers. Unfortunately, there is no single, agreed framework for synthesizing diverse forms of evidence. Approaches to synthesis will continue to be tested, developed and refined over the coming years, but it is to be hoped that this book has succeeded in outlining the kinds of methods currently available and suggested some ways that they might fruitfully be used, and potentially combined, to inform policy- and decision-making.

Useful reading

This is a guide to some of the key sources that provide further reading for those wishing to find out more about particular approaches and methods. It is not intended as an exhaustive guide, but lists a few key texts that readers may find useful.

Overviews of the synthesis of diverse evidence

Dixon-Woods, M. Agarwal, S., Young, B., Jones, D. and Sutton A. (2004) *Integrative Approaches to Qualitative and Quantitative Evidence*. London: Health Development Agency. http://www.nice.org.uk/page.aspx?o=508055.

Mays, N., Pope, C. and Popay, J. (2005) Systematically reviewing qualitative and quantitative evidence to inform management and policy-making in the health field. *Journal of Health Services Research and Policy*, 10(Suppl 1): 6–20.

Popay, J. (ed.) (2006) *Moving beyond Effectiveness in Evidence Synthesis: Methodological Issues in the Synthesis of Diverse Sources of Evidence*. London: National Institute of Health and Clinical Excellence.

Systematic review

NHS Centre for Reviews and Dissemination (2001) *Undertaking Systematic Reviews of Research on Effectiveness: CRD's Guidance for those Carrying out or Commissioning Reviews*, CRD report No. 4, 2nd edn. York: University of York. http://www.york.ac.uk/inst/crd/report4.htm.

Petticrew, M. and Roberts, H. (2006) *Systematic Reviews in the Social Sciences: A Practical Guide*. Oxford: Blackwell Publishing.

Quantitative approaches to synthesis

Cooper, N., Sutton, A. and Abrams, K. (2002) Decision analytic economic modelling within a Bayesian framework: application to prophylactic antibiotics' use for caesarean section. *Statistical Methods in Medical Research*, 11: 491–512.

Dowie, J. (2006) The Bayesian approach to decision-making, in A. Killoran, C. Swann and M. Kelly (eds) *Public Health Evidence: Tackling Health Inequalities*. Oxford: Oxford University Press, pp. 309–21.

Ragin, C.C. (1987) *The Comparative Method: Moving Beyond Qualitative and Quantitative Strategies*. Los Angeles, CA: University of California Press.

Roberts, K.A., Dixon-Woods, M., Fitzpatrick, R., Abrams, K.R. and Jones, D.R. (2002) Factors affecting uptake of childhood immunisation: a Bayesian synthesis of qualitative and quantitative evidence. *Lancet*, 360: 1596–9.

US General Accounting Office (1992) *Cross-design Synthesis: A New Strategy for Medical Effectiveness Research*. Washington, DC: General Accounting Office.

Yin, R., Heald, K. (1975) Using the case survey method to analyse policy studies. *Administrative Science Quarterly*, 20: 371–81.

Interpretive approaches to synthesis

Britten, N., Campbell, R., Pope, C., Donovan, J., Morgan, M. and Pill, R. (2002) Using meta ethnography to synthesize qualitative research: a worked example. *Journal of Health Services Research and Policy*, 7(4): 209–15.

Kearney, M. (2001) Enduring love: a grounded formal theory of women's experience of domestic violence. *Research in Nursing and Health*, 24: 270–82.

Noblit, G. and Hare, R. (1988) *Meta-ethnography: Synthesising Qualitative Studies*. Newbury Park, CA: Sage.

Mixed approaches to synthesis

Realist synthesis/meta-narrative mapping

Greenhalgh, T., Robert, G., Bate, P., Kyriakidou, O., Macfarlane, F. and Peacock, R. (2004) *Diffusion of Innovations in Health Service Organisations: A Systematic Literature Review*. Oxford: Blackwell Publishing.

Pawson, R. (2006) *Evidence-based Policy: A Realist Perspective*. London: Sage.

Narrative synthesis

Garcia, J., Bricker, L., Henderson, J., Martin, M-A., Mugford, M., Nielson, J. and Roberts, T. (2002) Women's views of pregnancy ultrasound: a systematic review. *Birth*, 29: 225–50.

Oliver, S., Harden, A., Rees, R., Shepherd, J., Brunton, G., Garcia, J. and Oakley, A. (2005) An emerging framework for including different types of evidence in systematic reviews for public policy. *Evaluation*, 11(4): 428–46.

Popay, J., Roberts, H., Sowden, A., Petticrew, M., Arai, L., Rodgers, M., Britten, N. (2006) *Guidance on the conduct of narrative synthesis in systematic reviews*. A product from the ESRC methods programme. Available from the Institute for Health Research, Lancaster University, UK.

Sequenced synthesis/EPPI Centre approach

Shepherd, J., Harden, A., Rees, R., Brunton, G., Garcia, J., Oliver, S. and Oakley, A. (2006) Young people and healthy eating: a systematic review of research on barriers and facilitators. *Health Education Research*, 21(2): 239–57.

References

Agranoff, R. and Radin, B.A. (1991) The comparative case study approach in public administration. *Research in Public Administration*, 1: 203–31.

Arai, L., Britten, N., Popay, J., Roberts, H., Petticrew, M., Rogers, M. and Sowden, A. Testing methodological developments in the conduct of narrative synthesis: a demonstration review. *Evidence and Policy* (forthcoming).

Attree, P. and Milton, B. (2006) Critically appraising qualitative research for systematic reviews: defusing the methodological cluster bombs. *Evidence and Policy*, 2(1): 109–26.

Barbour, R.S. (1999) The case for combining qualitative and quantitative methods in health services research. *Journal of Health Services Research and Policy*, 4: 39–43.

Black, N. (2001) Evidence based policy: proceed with care. *British Medical Journal*, 323: 275–8.

Black, N. (2006) Consensus development methods, in N. Mays and C. Pope (eds) *Qualitative Research in Health Care*, 3rd edn. Oxford: Blackwell Publishing/BMJ Books, pp. 132–41.

Black, N., Murphy, M., Lamping, D., McKee, M., Sanderson, C., Askham, J. and Marteau, T. (1998) Consensus development methods for creating clinical guidelines, in N. Black, J. Brazier, R. Fitzpatrick and B. Reeves (eds) *Health Services Research Methods: A Guide to Best Practice*. London: BMJ Books, pp. 199–211.

Black, N., Murphy, M., Lamping, D., McKee, M., Sanderson, C., Askham, J. and Marteau, T. (1999) Consensus development methods: a review of best practice in creating clinical guidelines. *Journal of Health Services Research and Policy*, 4(4): 236–48.

Bloor, M. (1997) Techniques of validation in qualitative research: a critical commentary, in G. Miller and R. Dingwall (eds) *Context and Method in Qualitative Research*. London: Sage, pp. 37–50.

Booth, A. (2004) Formulating answerable questions, in A. Booth and A. Brice (eds) *Evidence-based Practice for Information Professionals: A Handbook*. London: Facet, pp. 61–70.

Booth, A. and Fry-Smith, A. (2004) *Developing the Research Question*. Etext on Health Technology Assessment (HTA) Information Resources. http://www.nlm.nih.gov/archive//2060905/nichsr/ehta/chapter2.html (accessed 28 Oct. 2006).

Brannen, J. (1992) (ed.) *Mixing Methods: Qualitative and Quantitative Research*. Aldershot: Avebury.

Britten, N. (1996) Lay views of drugs and medicines: orthodox and unorthodox accounts, in S.J. Williams and M. Calnan (eds) *Modern Medicine. Lay Perspectives and Experiences*. London: UCL Press.

Britten, N., Campbell, R., Pope, C., Donovan, J., Morgan, M. and Pill, R. (2002) Using meta ethnography to synthesise qualitative research: a worked example. *Journal of Health Services Research and Policy*, 7(4): 209–15.

Bryman, A. (2004) *Social Research Methods*, 2nd edn. Oxford: Oxford University Press.

Burls, A., Cummins, C., Fry-Smith, A., Gold, L., Hyde, S.C., Jordan, R., Parry, D., Stevens, A., Wilson, R. and Young, J. (2000) *West Midlands Development and Evaluation Service Handbook*. Birmingham: West Midlands Development and Evaluation Service. http://www.pcpoh.bham.ac.uk/publichealth/wmhtac/pdf/wmhandbook.pdf (accessed 30 Oct. 2006).

Buse, K., Mays, N., Walt, G. (2005) *Making Health Policy*. Maidenhead: Open University Press.

Bushman, B. and Wells, G. (2001) Narrative impressions of literature: the availability bias and the corrective properties of meta-analytic approaches. *Personality and Social Psychology Bulletin*, 27: 1123–30.

Buzan, T. (1993) *The Mind Map Book. How to Use Radiant Thinking to Maximize Your Brain's Untapped Potential*. Harmondsworth: Penguin.

Campbell, R., Pound, P., Pope, C., Britten, N., Pill, R., Morgan, M. and Donovan, J. (2003) Evaluating meta-ethnography: a synthesis of qualitative research on lay experiences of diabetes and diabetes care. *Social Science and Medicine*, 56: 671–84.

Campbell, R., Pound, P., Morgan, M., Daker-White, G., Britten, N., Pill, R., Yardley, L., Pope, C. and Donovan, J. (forthcoming). Evaluating meta-ethnography: systematic anaylsis and synthesis: a qualitative research. Report for the National Coordinating Centre for Health Technology Assessment (NCCHTA).

Caracelli, V.J. and Riggin, L.J.C. (1994) Mixed-method evaluation: developing quality criteria through concept mapping. *Evaluation Practice*, 15: 139–52.

Casteel, C. and Peek-Asa, C. (2000) Effectiveness of crime prevention through environmental design (CPTED) in reducing robberies. *American Journal of Preventative Medicine*, 18(4 Suppl): 99–115.

Centers for Disease Control and Prevention (2005) *The Guide to Community Preventive Services: What Works to Promote Health*. Task force on community preventive services. Atlanta GA: CDC. http://thecommunityguide.org (accessed 29 Oct. 2006).

Chalmers, I. and Altman, D. (1995) (eds) *Systematic Reviews*. London: BMJ Books.

Chalmers, I., Enkin, M. and Keirse, M.J.N.C. (1989) *Effective Care in Pregnancy and Childbirth*. Oxford: Oxford University Press.

Chalmers, I., Enkin, M. and Kierse, M. (1993) Preparing and updating systematic reviews of randomised controlled trials of health care. *Milbank Quarterly*, 71: 411–37.

Chalmers, T., Smith, H., Blackburn, C., Silverman, B., Schroeder, B. and Reitman, D. (1981) A method for assessing the quality of a randomized controlled trial. *Controlled Clinical Trials*, 2: 31–49.

Clemmens, D. (2003) Adolescent motherhood: a meta-synthesis of qualitative Studies. *American Journal of Maternal Child Nursing*, 28(2): 93–9.

Clinkenbeard, P.R. (1991) Beyond summary: constructing a review of the literature, in N.K. Buchanan and J.F. Feldhusen (eds) *Conducting Research and Evaluation in Gifted Education: A Handbook of Methods and Applications*. New York: Teachers College Press, pp. 33–50.

Cochrane, A.L. (1972) *Effectiveness and Efficiency: Random Reflections on Health Services*. London: Nuffield Provincial Hospitals Trust (reprinted by RSM Press 1999).

Cooper, H. and Hedges, L. (eds) (1994) *The Handbook of Research Synthesis*. New York: Russell Sage Foundation.

Cooper, N., Sutton, A. and Abrams, K. (2002) Decision analytic economic modelling within a Bayesian framework: application to prophylactic antibiotics' use for caesarean section. *Statistical Methods in Medical Research*, 11: 491–512.

Curlette, W.L. and Cannella, K.S. (1985) Going beyond the narrative summarization of research findings: the meta-analysis approach. *Research in Nursing and Health*, 8: 293–301.

Cwikel, J., Behar, L. and Rabson-Hare, J. (2000) A comparison of a vote-count and meta-analysis review of intervention research with adult cancer patients. *Research on Social Work Practice*, 10: 139–58.

Davies, H.T.O., Nutley, S.M. and Smith, P.C. (2000) *What Works? Evidence-based Policy and Practice in Public Services*. Bristol: Policy Press.

Davies, P. (1999) What is evidence-based education? *British Journal of Educational Studies*, 47: 108–21.

Deeks, J., Khan, K.S., Song, F., Popay, J., Nixon, J. and Kleijnen, J. Data synthesis. In: Khan, K.S., ter Riet, G., Glanville, J., Sowden, A.J. and Kleignen, J., eds. *Undertaking systematic reviews of research on effectiveness: CRD's guidance for those carrying out or commissioning reviews*. York: NHS Centre for Reviews and Dissemination, University of York, 2001. Stage II, Phase 7, p. 18.

Denis, J-L. and Lomas, J. (eds) (2003) Researcher: decision-maker partnerships. *Journal of Health Services Research and Policy*, 8(Suppl 2): 1–6.

Dickersin, K., Scherer, R. and Lefebvre, C. (1994) Identifying relevant studies for systematic reviews. *British Medical Journal*, 309: 1286–91.

Dixon-Woods, M., Agarwal, S., Young, B., Jones, D. and Sutton, A. (2004) *Integrative Approaches to Qualitative and Quantitative Evidence*. London: Health Development Agency. http://www.nice.org.uk/page.aspx?o=508055 (accessed 17 Oct. 2006).

Dixon-Woods, M., Bonas, S., Booth, A., Jones, D.R., Miller, T., Sutton, A., Shaw, R., Smith, J. and Young, B. (2006a) How can systematic reviews incorporate qualitative research? A critical perspective. *Qualitative Research*, 6(1): 27–44.

Dixon-Woods, M., Cavers, D., Agarwal, S., Annandale, E., Arthur, A., Harvey, J., Hsu, R., Katbamna, S., Olsen, R., Smith, L.K., Riley, R. and Sutton, A. (2006b) Conducting critical interpretive synthesis of the literature on access to health-care by vulnerable groups. *BMC Research Methodology*, 6: 35.

Dixon-Woods, M., Fitzpatrick, R. and Roberts, K. (2001) Including qualitative research in systematic reviews: problems and opportunities. *Journal of Evaluation in Clinical Practice*, 7: 125–33.

Dixon-Woods, M. and Fitzpatrick, R. (2001) Qualitative research in systematic reviews has established a place for itself (editorial). *British Medical Journal*, 323: 765–66.

Dixon-Woods, M., Kirk, D., Agarwal, S., Annandale, E., Arthur, T., Harvey, J., Hsu, R., Katbamna, S., Olsen, R., Smith, L., Riley, R. and Sutton, A. (2005) *Vulnerable Groups and Access to Health Care: A Critical Interpretative Synthesis*. A report for the National Co-ordinating Centre for NHS Service Delivery and Organisation R and D (NCCSDO). http://www.sdo.lshtm.ac.uk/files/project/25-final-report.pdf (accessed 25 Oct. 2006).

Dowie, J. (2001) Towards value-based, science-informed public health policy: conceptual framework and practical guidelines. WHO/Department of Health Consultation on Risks to Health: Better Management for Decision-making.

Dowie, J. (2006) The Bayesian approach to decision-making, in A. Killoran, C. Swann and M. Kelly (eds) *Public Health Evidence: Tackling Health Inequalities*. Oxford: Oxford University Press, pp. 309–21.

Downs, S. and Black, N. (1998) The feasibility of creating a checklist for the assessment of the methodological quality of both randomised and non-randomised studies of healthcare interventions. *Journal of Epidemiology and Community Health*, 52: 377–84.

Doyle, L.H. (2003) Synthesis through meta-ethnography: paradoxes, enhancements, and possibilities. *Qualitative Research*, 3(3): 321–44.

Droitcour, J., Silberman, G. and Chelimsky, E. (1993) Cross-design synthesis: a new form of meta-analysis for combining results from randomised clinical trials and medical-practice databases. *International Journal of Technology Assessment in Health Care*, 9: 440–9.

Ekman, R. and Welander, G. (1998) The results of ten years' experience with the Skaraborg Bicycle Helmet Program in Sweden. *International Journal for Consumer and Product Safety*, 5(1): 23–39.

Estabrooks, C.A., Field, P.A. and Morse, J.M. (1994) Aggregating qualitative findings: an approach to theory development. *Qualitative Health Research*, 4: 503–11.

Erzberger, C. and Kelle, U. (2003) Making inferences in mixed methods: the rules of integration, in A. Tashakkori and C. Teddlie (eds) *Handbook of Mixed Methods in Social and Behavioural Research*. London: Sage, pp. 457–88.

Evans, D. (2002a) Database searches for qualitative research. *Journal of the Medical Library Association*, 90: 290–3.

Evans, D. (2002b) Systematic reviews of interpretive research: interpretive data synthesis of processed data. *Australian Journal of Advanced Nursing*, 20: 22–6.

Feder, G.S., Hutson, M., Ramsay, J. and Taket, A.R. (2006) Women exposed to intimate partner violence: expectations and experiences when they encounter health care professionals: a meta-analysis of qualitative studies. *Archives of Internal Medicine*, 166: 22–37.

Garcia, J., Bricker, L., Henderson, J., Martin, M-A., Mugford, M., Nielson, J. and Roberts, T. (2002) Women's views of pregnancy ultrasound: a systematic review. *Birth*, 29: 225–50.

Garratt, D. and Hodkinson, P. (1998) Can there be criteria for selecting research criteria? A hermeneutical analysis of an inescapable dilemma. *Qualitative Inquiry*, 4(4): 515–39.

Gibson, B. (2003) Beyond 'two communities', in V. Lin and B. Gibson (eds) *Evidence-based Health Policy: Problems and Possibilities*. Melbourne: Oxford University Press, pp. 18–30.

Glanville, J., Haines, M. and Auston, I. (1998) Finding information on clinical effectiveness. *British Medical Journal*, 317: 200–3.

Glaser, B. and Strauss, A. (1967) *The Discovery of Grounded Theory: Strategies for Qualitative Research*. Chicago: Aldine.

Glass, G., McGaw, B. and Smith, M. (1981) *Meta-analysis in Social Research*. Beverly Hills, CA: Sage.

Goodwin, N., Mays, N., McLeod, H., Malbon, G. and Raftery, J., on behalf of the Total Purchasing National Evaluation team (TP-NET) (1998) Evaluation of total purchasing pilots in England and Scotland and implications for primary care groups in England: personal interviews and analysis of routine data. *British Medical Journal*, 317: 256–9.

Grant, M.J. (2004) How does your searching grow? A survey of search preferences and the use of optimal search strategies in the identification of qualitative research. *Health Information and Libraries Journal*, 21(1): 21–32.

Grayson, L. and Gomersall, A. (2003) *A Difficult Business: Finding the Evidence for Social Science Reviews*. ESRC UK Centre for Evidence Based Policy and Practice, Working Paper 19. London: Department of Politics, Queen Mary College, University of London. http://www.evidencenetwork.org/Documents/wp19.pdf (accessed 27 Jul. 2004).

Greenhalgh, T., Robert, G., Bate, P., Kyriakidou, O., Macfarlane, F. and Peacock, R. (2004a) *Diffusion of Innovations in Health Service Organisations: A Systematic Literature Review*. Oxford: Blackwell Publishing.

Greenhalgh, T., Robert, G., Bate, P., Macfarlane, F. and Kyriakidou, C. (2004b) Diffusion of innovation in service organizations: systematic review and recommendations. *Milbank Quarterly*, 82(4): 581–629.

Greenhalgh, T., Robert, G., Macfarlane, F., Bate, S.P., Kyriakidou, O. and Peacock, R. (2005) Storylines of research in diffusion of innovation: a meta-narrative approach to systematic review. *Social Science and Medicine*, 61(2): 417–30.

Grimshaw, J., McAuley, L., Bero, L., Grilli, R., Oxman, A., Ramsay, C., et al. (2003) Systematic reviews of the effectiveness of quality improvement strategies and programmes. *Quality Safety Health Care*, 12: 298–303.

Haines, A., Kuruvilla, S. and Borchert, M. (2004) Bridging the implementation gap between knowledge and action for health. *Bulletin of the World Health Organization*. 82: 724–32.

Hammersley, M. (1992) *What's Wrong with Ethnography?* London: Routledge.

Hammersley, M. (2006) Systematic or unsystematic, is that the question? Some reflections on science, art and politics of reviewing research evidence, in A. Killoran, C. Swann and M. Kelly (eds) *Public Health Evidence: Tackling Health Inequalities*. Oxford: Oxford University Press, pp. 239–50.

Hammersley, M. and Atkinson, P. (1995) *Ethnography: Principles and Practice*, 2nd edn. London: Routledge.

Hanney, S., Gonzalez-Block, M., Buxton, M.J. and Kogan, M. (2003) The utilisation of health research in policy-making: concepts, examples and methods of assessment. *BMC Health Research Policy and Systems*, 1: 2.

Harden, A. and Thomas, J. (2005) Methodological issues in combining diverse study types in systematic reviews. *International Journal of Social Research Methodology*, 8(3): 257–71.

Harden, A., Garcia, J., Oliver, S., Rees, R., Shepherd, J., Brunton, G. and Oakley, A. (2004) Applying systematic review methods to studies of people's views: an example from public health research. *Journal of Epidemiology and Community Health*, 58: 794–800.

Harden, A., Oakley, A. and Oliver, S. (2001) Peer-delivered health promotion for young people: a systematic review of different study designs. *Health Education Journal*, 60: 1–15.

Hedges, L.V. and Olkin, I. (1985) *Statistical Methods for Meta-analysis*. London: Academic Press.

Hodson, R. (1999a) *Analyzing Documentary Accounts*. London: Sage.

Hodson, R. (1999b) Dignity in the workplace under participative management. *American Sociological Review*, 61: 719–38.

Hogan, B.E., Linden, W. and Najarian, B. (2002) Social support interventions: do they work? *Clinical Psychology Review*, 22: 381–440.

Howe, K.K. and Eisenhart, M. (1990) Standards for qualitative (and quantitative) research: a prolegomenon. *Educational Researcher*, 19(4): 2–9.

Hunter, J. and Schmidt, F. (2004) *Methods of Meta-analysis: Correcting Error and Bias in Research Findings*, 2nd edn. Newbury Park, CA: Sage.

Jadad, A. (1998) *Randomised Controlled Trials: A Users Guide*. London: BMJ Books.

Jailwala, J., Imperiale, T. and Kroenke, K. (2000) Pharmacologic treatment of the irritable bowel syndrome: a systematic review of randomised controlled trials. *Archives of Internal Medicine*, 33: 136–47.

Jensen, L.A. and Allen, M.N. (1994) A synthesis of qualitative research in wellness–illness. *Qualitative Health Research*, 4(4): 349–69.

Kearney, M. (2001) Enduring love: a grounded formal theory of women's experience of domestic violence. *Research in Nursing and Health*, 24: 270–82.

Kelly, M.P., Speller, V. and Meyrick J. (2004) *Getting Evidence into Practice in Public Health*. London: Health Development Agency. http://www.nice.org.uk/page.aspx?o=508124 (accessed 17 Oct. 2006).

Khan, K., ter Reit, G., Popay, J., Nixon, J. and Kleijnen, J. (2001) Phase 5: Study quality assessment, in *NHS Centre for Reviews and Dissemination. Undertaking Systematic Reviews of Research on Effectiveness: CRD's Guidance for those Carrying out or Commissioning Reviews*, CRD Report No. 4, 2nd edn. York: University of York. http://www.york.ac.uk/inst/crd/pdf/crd4_ph5.pdf (accessed 30 Oct. 2007).

Kingdon, J.W. (1997) *Agendas, Alternatives and Public Policies*, 2nd edn. New York: Longman.

Klassen, T.P., Mackay, J.M., Moher, D., Walker, A. and Jones, A.L. (2000) Community-based injury prevention interventions. *Unintentional Injuries in Childhood*, 10(1): 83–110.

Konno, R. (2006) Support for overseas qualified nurses in adjusting to Australian nursing practice: a systematic review. *International Journal of Evidenced-based Healthcare*, 2: 83–100.

Kvale, S. (1996) *InterViews: an Introduction to Qualitative Research Interviewing*. Thousand Oaks, CA: Sage.

Lamarche, P.A., Beaulieu, M-D., Pineault, R., Contandriopoulos, A-P., Denis, J-L. and Haggerty, J. (2003) Choices for change: the path for restructuring primary healthcare services in Canada. Report submitted to the partners: Canadian Health Services Research Foundation, New Brunswick Department of Health and Wellness, Saskatchewan Department of Health, Ministère de la santé et des services sociaux du Québec and Health Canada. Ottawa: Canadian Health Services Research Foundation. http://www.chsrf.ca/final_research/commissioned_research/policy_synthesis/pdf/choices_for_change_e.pdf (accessed 17 Oct. 2006).

Larsson, R. (1993) Case survey methodology: quantitative analysis of patterns across case studies. *Academy of Management Journal*, 36(6): 1515–46.

Lavis, J., Davies, H., Oxman, A., Denis, J-L., Golden-Biddle, K. and Ferlie, E. (2005) Towards systematic reviews that inform health care management and policy-making. *Journal of Health Services Research and Policy*, 10(Suppl 1): 35–48.

Lavis, J., Ross, S., McLeod, C. and Gildner, A. (2003) Measuring the impact of health research. *Journal of Health Services Research and Policy*, 8(3): 165–70.

Lewis, J., Spencer, L., Ritchie, J. and Dillon, L. (2006) Appraising quality in qualitative evaluations: approaches and challenges, in J. Popay (ed.) *Moving beyond Effectiveness in Evidence Synthesis: Methodological Issues in the Synthesis of Diverse Sources of Evidence*. London: National Institute of Health and Clinical Excellence.

Light, R.J. and Pillemer, D.B. (1984) *Summing Up: The Science of Reviewing Research*. Cambridge, MA: Harvard University Press.

Lin, V. (2003) Improving the research and policy partnership: an agenda for research transfer and governance, in V. Lin and B. Gibson (eds) *Evidence-based Health Policy: Problems and Possibilities*. Melbourne: Oxford University Press, pp. 285–97.

Lin, V. and Gibson, B. (eds) (2003) *Evidence-based Health Policy: Problems and Possibilities*. Melbourne: Oxford University Press.

Lincoln, Y.S. and Guba, E.G. (1985) *Naturalistic Enquiry*. Newbury Park, CA: Sage.

Lindblom, C.E. (1990) *Inquiry and Change: The Troubled Attempt to Understand and Shape Society*. New Haven, CT: Yale University Press.

Lloyd Jones, M. (2005) Role development and effective practice in specialist and advanced practice roles in acute hospital settings: systematic review and meta-synthesis. *Journal of Advanced Nursing*, 49(2): 191–209.

Lomas, J. (2000) Connecting research and policy. Isuma: *Canadian Journal of Policy Research*, 1: 140–4.

Lomas, J., Culyer, A., McCutcheon, C., McAuley, L. and Law, S. (2005) *Conceptualizing and Combining Evidence for Health System Guidance*. Ottawa: Canadian Health Services Research Foundation.

Luce, B.R., Claxton, K. (1999) Redefining the analytical approach to pharmacoeconomics. *Health Economics*, 8(3): 187–9.

Lumme-Sandt, K., Hervonen, A. and Jylha, M. (2000) Interpretative repertoires of medicine among the oldest-old. *Social Science and Medicine*, 50: 1843–50.

McCormick, J., Rodney, P. and Varcoe, C. (2003) Reinterpretation across studies: an approach to meta-analysis. *Qualitative Health Research*, 13(7): 933–44.

McNaughton, D.B. (2000) A synthesis of qualitative home visiting research. *Public Health Nursing*, 17(6): 405–14.

Martin, M. (2005) The need for an overall strategy. *Journal of Health Service Research and Policy*, 10(Supp 1): 49–50.

Mayor, S. (2001) Row over breast cancer screening shows that scientists bring 'some subjectivity' into their work. *British Medical Journal*, 323: 956.

Mays, N. and Pope, C. (2006) Quality in qualitative health research, in C. Pope and N. Mays (eds) *Qualitative Research in Health Care*, 3rd edn. Oxford: Blackwell Publishing/BMJ Books, pp. 82–101.

Mays, N., Pope, C. and Popay, J. (2005) Systematically reviewing qualitative and quantitative evidence to inform management and policy-making in the health field. *Journal of Health Services Research and Policy*, 10(Suppl 1): 6–20.

Melchart, D., Linde, K., Fischer, P., Berman, B., White, A., Vickers, A. and Allais, G. (2004) *Acupuncture for Idiopathic Headache* (Cochrane Review), in the Cochrane Library, Issue 3. Chichester: John Wiley & Sons.

Miles, M.B. and Huberman, A.M. (1994) *Qualitative Data Analysis: An Expanded Sourcebook*. London: Sage.

Miller, D. and Reilly, J. (1995) Making an issue of food safety: the media, pressure groups and the public sphere, in D. Maurer and J. Sobal (eds) *Food and Nutrition as Social Problems*. New York: Aldine de Gruyter.

Mintzberg, H., Raisinghani, D. and Theoret, A. (1976) The structure of 'unstructured' decision processes. *Administrative Science Quarterly* 21: 246–75.

Mitton, C. and Patten, S. (2004) Evidence-based priority setting: what do decision-makers think? *Journal of Health Services Research and Policy*, 9: 146–52.

Moher, D., Schulz, K.F. and Altman, D.G. (2001) The CONSORT statement: revised recommendations for improving the quality of reports of parallel group randomized trials. *BMC Medical Research Methodology*, 1: 2.

Moore, B. (1966) *Social Origins of Dictatorship and Democracy: Lord and Peasant in the Making of the Modern World*. Boston: Beacon Press.

Mulrow, C. and Cook, D. (1998) *Systematic Reviews: Synthesis of Best Evidence for Health Care Decisions*. Philadelphia: American College of Physicians.

Mulrow, C., Langhorne, P. and Grimshaw, J. (1998) Integrating heterogeneous pieces of evidence in systematic reviews, in C. Mulrow and D. Cook (eds) *Systematic Reviews: Synthesis of Best Evidence for Healthcare Decisions*. Philadelphia: American College of Physicians, pp. 103–12.

Murphy, E., Dingwall, R., Greatbach, D., Parker, S. and Watson, P. (1998) Qualitative research methods in health technology assessment: a review of the literature. *Health Technology Assessment*, 2(16).

NHS Centre for Reviews and Dissemination (2001) *Undertaking Systematic Reviews of Research on Effectiveness: CRD's Guidance for those Carrying out or Commissioning Reviews*, CRD Report No. 4, 2nd edn. York: University of York. http://www.york.ac.uk/inst/crd/report4.htm.

Noblit, G. and Hare, R. (1988) *Meta-ethnography: Synthesising Qualitative Studies*. Newbury Park, CA: Sage.

Nutley, S. and Webb, J. (2000) Evidence and the policy process, in H.T.O Davies, S.M. Nutley and P.C. Smith (eds) *What works? Evidence-based Policy and Practice in Public Services*. Bristol: Policy Press, pp. 13–41.

O'Cathain, A. and Thomas, K. (2006) Combining qualitative and quantitative methods, in C. Pope and N. Mays (eds) *Qualitative Research in Health Care*, 3rd edn. Oxford: Blackwell Publishing/BMJ Books, pp. 102–11.

Oliver, S., Harden, A., Rees, R., Shepherd, J., Brunton, G., Garcia, J. and Oakley, A. (2005) An emerging framework for including different types of evidence in systematic reviews for public policy. *Evaluation*, 11(4): 428–46.

Oliver, S., Oakley, L., Lumley, J. and Waters, E. (2001) Smoking cessation programmes in pregnancy: systematically addressing development, implementation, women's concerns and effectiveness. *Health Education Journal*, 60: 362–70.

Olsen, O. and Gøtzche, P.C. (2001) Cochrane review on screening for breast cancer with ammnography. *Lancet*, 358: 1340–4.

Paterson, B.L., Thorne, S., Canam, C. and Jillings, C. (2001) *Meta-study of Qualitative*

Health Research: A Practical Guide to Meta-analysis and Meta-synthesis. Thousand Oaks, CA: Sage.

Paterson, B.L., Thorne, S. and Dewis, M. (1998) Adapting to and managing diabetes: image. *Journal of Nursing Scholarship*, 30(1): 57–62.

Pawson, R. (2002) Evidence-based policy: in search of a method. *Evaluation*, 8(2): 157–81.

Pawson, R. (2006) *Evidence-based Policy: A Realist Perspective.* London: Sage.

Pawson, R. and Bellaby, P. (2006) Realist synthesis: an explanatory focus for systematic review, in J. Popay (ed.) *Putting Effectiveness into Context: Methodological Issues in the Synthesis of Evidence from Diverse Study Designs.* London: Health Development Agency, pp. 83–94.

Pawson, R., Greenhalgh, T., Harvey, G. and Walshe, K. (2005) Realist review – a new method of systematic review designed for complex policy interventions. *Journal of Health Services Research and Policy*, 10(Suppl 1): 21–34.

Petticrew, M. and Roberts, H. (2005) Evidence, hierarchies, and typologies: horses for courses. *Journal of Epidemiology and Community Health*, 57: 527–9.

Petticrew, M. and Roberts, H. (2006) *Systematic Reviews in the Social Sciences: A Practical Guide.* Oxford: Blackwell Publishing.

Pielstick, C.D. (1998) The transforming leader: a meta-ethnographic analysis. *Community College Review*, 26(3): 15–34.

Popay, J., Rogers, A. and Williams, G. (1998) Rationale and standards for the systematic review of qualitative literature in health services research. *Qualitative Health Research*, 8: 341–51.

Popay, J. and Williams, G. (1998) Qualitative Research and Evidence Based Health care. *Journal of the Royal Society of Medicine*, 91(Suppl. 35): 32–7.

Popay, J., Roberts, H., Sowden, A., Petticrew, M., Arai, L., Rodger, M., Britten, N., with Roen, K., Duffy, S. (2006) Guidance on the conduct of narrative synthesis in systematic reviews. Version 3. A product from the ESRC methods programme. Available from the Institute for Health Research, Lancaster University, UK.

Pope, C. (2003) Resisting evidence: contemporary social movements in medicine. *Health*, 7: 267–82.

Pope, C. and Mays, N. (1993) Opening the black box: an encounter in the corridors of health services research. *British Medical Journal*, 306: 315–18.

Pope, C. and Mays, N. (2006) *Qualitative Research in Health Care.* Oxford: Blackwell Publishing/BMJ Books.

Popper, K. (1959) *The Logic of Scientific Discovery.* London: Hutchinson.

Pound, P., Britten, N., Morgan, M., Yardley, L., Pope, C., Daker-White, G. and Campbell, R. (2005) Resisting medicines: a synthesis of qualitative studies of medicine taking. *Social Science and Medicine*, 61: 133–55.

Ragin, C.C. (1987) *The Comparative Method: Moving beyond Qualitative and Quantitative Strategies.* Los Angeles, CA: University of California Press.

Rice, E.H. (2002) The collaboration process in professional development schools results of a meta-ethnography 1990–1998. *Journal of Teacher Education*, 53(1): 55–67.

Riley, T., Hawe, P. and Shiell, A. (2005) Contested ground: how should qualitative evidence inform the conduct of a community intervention trial? *Journal of Health Services Research and Policy*, 10: 103–10.

Ritchie, J. and Lewis, J (2003). *Qualitative Research Practice: A Guide for Social Science Students and Researchers*. London: Sage.

Roberts, K.A., Dixon-Woods, M., Fitzpatrick, R., Abrams, K.R. and Jones, D.R. (2002) Factors affecting uptake of childhood immunisation: a Bayesian synthesis of qualitative and quantitative evidence. *Lancet*, 360: 1596–9.

Rutter, M., Maughan, B., Mortimore, P. and Ouston, J. (1998) *Anti-social Behaviour by Young People*. Cambridge: Cambridge University Press.

Sabatier, P.A. and Jenkins-Smith, H.C. (1993) *Policy Change and Learning: An Advocacy Coalition Approach*. Boulder, CO: Westview Press.

Sandelowski, M., Docherty, S. and Emden, C. (1997) Qualitative metasynthesis: issues and techniques. *Research in Nursing and Health*, 20: 365–71.

Schreiber, R., Crooks, D. and Stern, P.N. (1997) Qualitative meta-analysis, in J.M. Morse (ed.) *Completing a Qualitative Project: Details and Dialogue*. Thousand Oaks, CA: Sage.

Schutz, A. (1962) *Collected Papers*, Vol. 1. The Hague: Nijhoff.

Schwarz, D.F., Grisso, J.A., Miles, C., Holmes, J.H. and Sutton, R.L. (1993) An injury prevention program in an urban African-American community. *American Journal of Public Health*, 83(5): 675–80.

Seale, S. and Silverman, D. (1997) Ensuring rigour in qualitative research. *European Journal of Public Health*, 7: 389–4.

Shadish, W., Cook, T. and Leviton, L. (1991) *Foundations of Program Evaluation*. Newbury Park, CA: Sage.

Shaw, R.L., Booth, A., Sutton, A.J., Miller, T., Smith, J.A., Young, B., Jones, D.R. and Dixon-Woods, M. (2004) Finding qualitative research: an evaluation of search strategies. *BMC Medical Research Methodology*, 4: 5.

Sheldon, T. (2005) Making evidence synthesis more useful for management and policy-making. *Journal of Health Services Research and Policy*, 10(Suppl 1): 1–5.

Shepherd, J., Harden, A., Rees, R., Brunton, G., Garcia, J., Oliver, S. and Oakley, A. (2006) Young people and healthy eating: a systematic review of research on barriers and facilitators. *Health Education Research*, 21 (2): 239–57.

Siau, K. and Long, Y. (2005) Synthesizing e-government stage models – a meta-synthesis based on meta-ethnography approach. *Industrial Management and Data Systems*, 105(4): 443–58.

Slavin, R.E. (1995) Best evidence synthesis: an intelligent alternative to meta-analysis. *Journal of Clinical Epidemiology*, 48: 9–18.

Smith, L., Pope, C. and Botha, J. (2005) Patients' help-seeking experiences and delay in cancer presentation: a qualitative synthesis. *Lancet*, 366: 825–31.

Solesbury, W. (2001) Evidence-based policy: whence it came from and where it's going. ESRC Centre for Evidence-based Policy and Practice working paper. http://www.evidencenetwork.co.uk/Documents/wp1.pdf (accessed 27 Oct. 2006).

Spencer, L., Ritchie, J., Lewis, J. and Dillon, L. (2003) *Quality in Qualitative Evaluation: A Framework for Assessing Research Evidence*. London: Government Chief Social Researcher's Office, Prime Minister's Strategy Unit, Cabinet Office. http://www.policyhub.gov.uk/evaluating_policy/qual_eval.asp (accessed 17 Oct. 2006).

Spiegelhalter, D.J., Myles, J.P., Jones, D.R. and Abrams, K.R. (2000) Bayesian methods in health technology assessment: a review. *Health Technology Assessment*, 4(38).

Stemler, S. (2001) An overview of content analysis. *Practical Assessment, Research and Evaluation*, 7(17) http://PAREonline.net/getvn.asp?v=7andn=17 (accessed 29 Oct. 2006).

Strauss, A.L. and Corbin, J. (1990) *Basics of Qualitative Research: Techniques and Procedures for Developing Grounded Theory*. Thousand Oaks, CA: Sage.

Suri, H. (2000) A critique of contemporary methods of research synthesis. *Post-Script*, 1: 49–55.

Svanström, L., Schelp, L., Robert, E. and Lindström, Å. (1996) Falköping, Sweden, ten years after: still a safe community? *International Journal for Consumer Safety*, 3(1): 1–7.

Thomas, J., Harden, A., Oakley, A., Oliver, S., Sutcliffe, K., Rees, R., Brunton, G. and Kavanagh, J. (2004) Integrating qualitative research with trials in systematic reviews. *British Medical Journal*, 328: 1010–12.

Turner, D., Wailoo, A., Nicholson, K., Cooper, N., Sutton, A. and Abrams, K. (2003) Systematic review and economic decision modelling for the prevention and treatment of influenza A and B. *Health Technology Assessment*, 7(35).

US General Accounting Office (1992) *Cross-design Synthesis: A New Strategy for Medical Effectiveness Research*. Washington, DC: General Accounting Office.

Van Maanen, J. (1988) *Tales of the Field: On Writing Ethnography*. Chicago: Chicago University Press.

Walter, F., Emery, J., Braithwaite, D. and Marteau, T. (2004) Lay understanding of familial risk of common chronic diseases: a systematic review and synthesis of qualitative research. *Annals of Family Medicine*, 2: 583–94.

Weiss, C.H. (1979) The many meanings of research utilization. *Public Administration Review*, 39: 426–31.

Weiss, C.H. (1986) The circuitry of enlightenment: diffusion of social science research to policy-makers. *Knowledge: Creation, Diffusion, Utilization*, 8: 274–81.

Weiss, C.H. (1991) Policy research: data, ideas or arguments?, in P. Wagner, C.H. Weiss, B. Wittrock and H. Wollmann (eds) *Social Sciences and Modern States*. Cambridge: Cambridge University Press, pp. 307–32.

White, C., Woodfield, K. and Ritchie, J. (2003) Reporting and presenting qualitative data, in J. Ritche and J. Lewis (eds) *Qualitative Research Practice*. London: Sage.

Yin, R. (1984) *Case Study Research, Design and Methods*, Applied Social Research Methods Series, Vol. 5. Thousand Oaks, CA: Sage.

Yin, R.K. (1986) Community crime prevention: a synthesis of eleven evaluations, in D.P. Rosenbaum (ed.) *Community Crime Prevention: Does it Work?* Sage Criminal Justice System Annuals, Vol. 22. Beverly Hills, CA: Sage, pp. 294–308.

Yin, R. and Heald, K. (1975) Using the case survey method to analyse policy studies. *Administrative Science Quarterly*, 20: 371–81.

Yin, R. and Yates, D. (1975) *Street-level Governments: Assessing Decentralization and Urban Services.* Lexington, MA: D.C. Heath.

Ytterstad, B. and Wasmuth, H. (1995) The Harstad Injury Prevention Study: evaluation of hospital-based injury recording and community-based intervention for traffic injury prevention. *Accident, Analysis and Prevention*, 27(1): 111–23.

Ytterstad, B., Smith, G.S. and Coggan, C.A. (1998) Harstad Injury Prevention Study: prevention of burns in young children by community-based intervention. *Injury Prevention*, 4(3): 176–80.

Index

ACF (advocacy coalition framework), 167–8
aggregative synthesis, 16, 17
Agranoff, R., 78, 79
anecdotal reports, 12, 13
assessment of study quality *see* quality
    appraisal
Atlas-Ti software, 135
axial coding, and grounded theory, 77

Bayesian approaches, 48, 55–67, 71, 173
    applying to synthesis, 56–7
    and cross-design synthesis, 59
    implications of, 57–9
    strengths and limitations of, 66–7
    to comprehensive decision modelling,
        64–5
    to meta-analysis, 48, 55, 60–2, 179
Bellaby, P., 8–9, 97, 98, 99–100
Best Evidence Synthesis (BES), 110
bias, in first generation literature reviews, 5
Black, N., 157
Boolean analysis, 47, 48
Brannen, J., 41
Britten, N., 83, 110

Campbell Collaboration, 10, 11, 24
Caracelli and Riggin, 181
case-controlled studies, 12
causality, configuration approach to, 8–9
charts, 128
    radar charts, 131–3
CHSRF (Canadian Health Services Research
        Foundation), 151, 165
    report format, 137, 141, 142–3
Clinkenbeard, P.R., 126–8
Cochrane Collaboration, 10, 11, 13, 22, 24,
        28, 30
    systematic reviews, 10, 97, 102, 137
cohort studies, 12
comparative analysis, 67–70, 96
comparative approaches, to interpretive
        synthesis, 76–9
comparative case studies, 78–9
comparative synthesis methods, 45

comprehensive decision modelling
    Bayesian approach to, 64–5
    and cross-design synthesis, 59
comprehensive literature searching, 29–31
computer software
    for content analysis, 50, 51
    and data extraction, 42
    producing Kiviat/radar charts, 133
    to support synthesis and reviewing, 136–7
conceptual mapping, 109, 127–9
content analysis, 48–51, 71, 96, 108
    computer software for, 50, 51
    defining, 48–9
    strengths and limitations of, 50
context-bound research, 3–4
Cooper, H., 60
cost-effectiveness analysis, 55
    Bayesian approaches to, 62–4
    and cross-design synthesis, 59
critical appraisal *see* quality appraisal
critical interpretive synthesis, 79, 86–7
cross-case analysis, 73
cross-design synthesis, 59

data dredging, 105
data extraction, 41–3
    summarising, 120
Davies, P., 162
decision analysis, 48
decision modelling, 55
decision support reviews, 13–15, 19–21,
        162–3, 173, 174, 192, 184
decision-makers *see* policy-makers
Delphi consensus exercise, 132
discriminant analysis, 70
disparate evidence, and synthesis, 17–18
dissemination of systematic reviews, 44
diverse evidence, quality appraisal of, 54
Dixon-Woods, M., 8, 16, 45, 86, 87, 93, 102,
        136, 151
Dowie, J., 65
Doyle, L.H., 87

EBM (evidence-based medicine), 153

effectiveness reviews, 9–12
  evidence hierarchy for, 12–13, 26–7
  knowledge support versus decision support
    reviews, 13–15
  quality appraisal, 32
electronic databases, 29–31
electronic search strategies, 119–20
engineering model, of evidence-policy
    relationships, 156
enlightenment model, of evidence-policy
    relationships, 155–8
EPPI approach to evidence review, 95–6,
    106–14, 150, 178–9
  main steps in, 112
  meta-synthesis matrix, 111, 113
  strengths and limitations of, 114
Erzberger, C., 179
ESRC (Economic and Social Research
    Council), 103
ethnography, 72, 151
  see also meta-ethnography
evidence synthesis see synthesis
evidence-based medicine (EBM), 153
evidence-based policy, 153
evidence-policy relationships, 155–64
  building, 163–4
  engineering model of, 156
  enlightenment model of, 155–8
  making the review relevant, 162–3
  reducing gap between research and policy,
    160–1
  timeliness in, 163
  two communities model of, 158–62, 165,
    168, 170
exploratory mapping, and second generation
    literature reviews, 7

falsification theory, and realist synthesis, 98
first generation literature reviews, 4–5, 8
  and narrative synthesis, 103
  and realist synthesis, 97, 101
  thematic analysis of, 96, 97
forest plots, and narrative synthesis, 108
frequency distributions, and narrative
    synthesis, 108
funnel plots, 109, 131

Gibson, B., 165–6, 168–9
Glaser, B., 76, 78
graphs
  graphical presentations, 131–2

and narrative synthesis, 108
Greenhalgh, T., 6–8, 44, 133–4
'grey' (unpublished) literature, 3
  searches for, 24, 29
grounded theory, 75, 76–9, 88, 93
  strengths and limitations of, 79

Hammersley, M., 16, 17
Harden, A., 24–5, 110
Hare, R., 6, 16, 79–81, 82, 83, 84
Heald, K., 55
Hedges, L., 60
hierarchies of evidence, 12–13, 26–7, 31
'higher order' synthesis, 95, 96
Hodson, R., 48, 49–50
Hogan, B.E., 121
Huberman, A.M., 88, 89, 93

idea webbing, 110, 126–7
illness maps, 84–5
individual studies, data extraction from, 41
information technology, 4
integrative synthesis, 16, 178–9
internet
  literature searches, 29
  World Wide Web, 3, 4
    Web reports, 140–1
interpretive synthesis, 16, 43, 45, 72–94, 192,
    178, 179
  combining qualitative and quantitative
    evidence, 73–4, 93–4
  comparative approaches to, 76–9
  data extraction, 41
  feasibility of synthesising qualitative
    evidence, 74–5
  presentation of, 151
  techniques for comparing studies in,
    88–93
  terminology, 75–6
  translation-based approaches to, 79–93
  understanding qualitative research
    methods, 72–3
  see also meta-ethnography

Joanna Briggs Institute, 29, 33, 136
  Qualitative Assessment and Review
    Instrument, 33
Joseph Rowntree Foundation, 'Findings'
    briefings, 163, 148–9
journal papers, 139
  style issues, 137–8

Kearney, M., 77–8
Kelle, U., 179
Kiviat diagrams, 131–3
knowledge support reviews, 13–15, 19–21,
    162–3, 174, 192
knowledge synthesis, 80
knowledge transfer, 151

L'Abbé plots, and narrative synthesis, 109
Lavis, J., 162, 163
Lin, V., 158
line of argument synthesis, and meta-
    ethnography, 81, 82, 84
linear systematic reviews, 19
    and synthesis, 16, 17
linkage and exchange movement, 158–62,
    165
literature reviews
    and aggregative synthesis, 16
    first generation, 4–5, 8, 96, 97, 101, 103
    second generation, 6–8, 184
    strengths and limitations of, 8–9
literature searching, 29–31, 119–20
Lloyd Jones, M., 88–93, 97
log-linear analysis, 70
logical (Boolean) analysis, 47
Lomas, J., 155
Lumme-Sandt, K., 85
lumping approach to systematic reviews, 27,
    28

McCormick, J., 75
McNaughton, D.B., 88, 93
mapping review questions, 23–4
matrices
    displaying information in, 127, 130
    and interpretive synthesis, 88–93
Mays, N., 181
meta-analysis, 11–12, 16, 173
    Bayesian approaches to, 48, 55, 60–2, 179
    and narrative synthesis, 102–3
    qualitative, 75
    of quantitative case surveys, 53
meta-ethnography, 6, 33, 42, 43, 73, 75–6,
    79–88, 93, 192
    assessing quality of, 181
    and critical interpretive synthesis, 86–7
    defining, 79–80
    of medicine-taking, 83–6
    and mixed methods synthesis, 95
    and narrative synthesis, 102, 103, 109

presentation of final synthesis results,
    133–4
stages of, 80–3
strengths and limitations of, 87–8
and thematic analysis, 96
meta-synthesis, 75
Miles, M.B., 88, 89, 93
Miller, D., 49
Mintzberg, H., 157–8
mixed methods synthesis, 95–114, 171–2,
    173, 177–8, 181
    EPPI approach to combining separate
        syntheses, 95–6, 106–14
    narrative synthesis, 95, 102–6, 107–10,
        114
    realist synthesis, 95, 97–101, 114
    thematic analysis, 95, 96–7, 108
    use of software in, 136
moderator variables, and narrative synthesis,
    107
Mulrow, C., 127, 128
multiple case study methods, 79
Murphy, E., 54

narrative synthesis, 95, 102–6, 114, 173, 192
    and data dredging, 105
    defining, 102–3
    main elements in, 104
    strengths and limitations of, 103–5
    tools and techniques for, 105–6, 107–10
NHS
    Centre for Reviews and Dissemination, 33,
        102
    Service Delivery and Organisation
        Research and Development Programme,
        151
Noblit, G., 6, 16, 79–81, 82, 83, 84
notes, organising and structuring, 118–19

O'Cathain, A., 179
oral presentations, 139
organisational innovations
    literature review on, 6–8, 43
    reports for policy- and decision-makers,
        141–7
Oxford Centre for Evidence-Based Medicine,
    grading system, 31

Pawson, R., 8–9, 97, 98, 99–100, 158, 162,
    169
Petticrew, M., 118

PICO framework for developing review
  questions, 24, 29
Plain English Campaign, 137
planning presentation, 118–20
policy brokers, 168
policy communities, 166–7, 168–9
policy networks, 166–7, 170
policy-makers, 153–70
  and the ACF (advocacy coalition
    framework), 167–8
  choice of research method for
    policy/decision-making, 171–2
  implications of the Bayesian approach for,
    57–9
  reports for, 141–7
  and systematic reviews, 153–4
  see also evidence-policy relationships
Popay, J., 103, 104, 105
Pope, C., 181
Popper, K., 98
positivism, 74
Pound, P., 44, 84, 85
proximal similarity of literature reviews, 9
published literature, 3

QSR software, 135
qualitative comparative analysis, 48, 67–70
  strengths and limitations of, 70
qualitative meta-analysis, 75
qualitative research evidence, 12, 13, 16
  assessing quality of reviews of, 180–2
  Bayesian meta-analysis of, 60–2
  data extraction from, 41
  quality appraisal of, 32–3, 54
  searching for, 30
  synthesis, 16, 17–18, 42–3, 46, 172, 173
    and content analysis, 49–50
    issues in reporting, 147–9
  systematic reviews of, 23, 28, 47–8
  thematic analysis of, 96
  see also interpretive synthesis
qualitative synthesis methods, 45
  text-based, 46
quality appraisal, 31–40
  of diverse evidence, 54
  effectiveness reviews, 32
  example of, 33–40
  of first generation literature reviews, 5
  of qualitative research, 32–3, 54
quantitative case surveys, 48, 51–5, 71
  strengths and limitations of, 54–5

quantitative content analysis, 48–51, 71
quantitative research evidence, 12, 13
  assessing quality of reviews of, 180–2
  data extraction, 41
  and interpretive synthesis, 73–4
  synthesis, 16, 18, 42–3, 46, 47–71, 172,
    173, 178
    Bayesian approach to, 48, 55–67, 71
    and qualitative comparative analysis,
      67–70, 71
    and triangulation, 180
  systematic reviews of, 23
  thematic analysis of, 96
quantitative synthesis methods, 45, 47–71
quantitative trials, Bayesian approach to,
  56–7
questions see review questions

radar charts, 131–3
Radin, B.A., 78, 79
Ragin, C.C., 67–8, 70
randomised controlled trials (RCTs), 3, 10,
  12, 28, 184
  Bayesian approaches to, 66
  and cross-design synthesis, 59
  and evidence-based medicine, 153
  inclusion criteria, 31
  and meta-analysis, 60
  and meta-ethnography, 80
  searching for, 30
  and synthesis, 42
realist synthesis, 6, 27, 95, 97–101, 114, 173
  data extraction, 41
  defining, 97–8
  miniature example of, 98–9
  of peer support, 99–101
  strengths and weaknesses of, 101
reciprocal translation, and meta-
  ethnography, 81, 84–6
record keeping
  notes, 118–19
  searches, 119–20
  synthesis process, 120
refutational synthesis, and meta-
  ethnography, 81–2
Reilly, J., 49
relationships, techniques for displaying and
  exploring, 126–33
resistance, and the meta-ethnography of
  medicine-taking, 86
review questions, 22–6

and data extraction, 41
RevMan software, 42, 137
Riley, T., 180
Roberts, H., 118
Rutter, M., 5–6, 8
RWJF (Robert Wood Johnson Foundation),
    Synthesis Project, 141, 144–7

Salford University Public Health Resource
    Unit, Critical Appraisal Tool, 33
sampling, and systematic reviews of
    effectiveness, 27–8
Sandelowski, M., 74
Schutz, A., 83–4
second generation literature reviews, 6–8,
    184
second order interpretations, meta-
    ethnography of medicine-taking, 84–5
selective coding, and grounded theory, 77–8
Shadish, W., 9
Sheldon, T., 154
Slavin, R.E., 110
Social Origins of Dictatorship and Democracy
    (Moore), 78
Solesbury, W., 153
Spencer, L., 181
SPICE framework for developing review
    questions, 24, 29
Spiegelhalter, D.J., 56
splitting approach to systematic reviews, 27
statistical meta-analysis, 42, 80
statistical presentations, 130–1
Stemler, S., 48
Strauss, A., 76, 78
subjective judgement, and Bayesian theory,
    56–7
substantive coding, and grounded theory, 77
SUMARI software, 29, 42, 136
Suri, H., 126
synthesis, 15–18, 42–3
    case for, 184–5
    choosing and combining approaches to,
        171–80
    cross-design, 59
    and data extraction, 41
    defining, 16
    and disparate evidence, 17–18
    organisation and presentation, 117–52
        exploring and displaying relationships,
            126–33
        final synthesis results/theories, 133–5

journal papers, 137–8, 140
    oral presentations, 139
    planning presentation, 118–20
    qualitative synthesis reports, 147–9
    qualitative-quantitative synthesis, 150
    reasons for, 117
    recording the searches, 119–20
    reports, 138–41
    style and voice, 137–8
    visual displays of synthesis material,
        121–26
    Web reports, 140–1
    programmes of, 164
    and quality appraisal, 31–40
    quantitative, 16, 18, 42–3, 46, 47–71
    typology of, 16
    see also interpretive synthesis; mixed
        methods synthesis
systematic reviews, 9–12, 13, 19–43, 74
    and aggregative synthesis, 16
    comprehensive literature searching, 29–31
    and data extraction, 40–2
    and decision support, 13–15, 19–21
    defining the question/questions, 22–6
    determining types of study to be included,
        26–9
    dissemination of, 43
    and evidence-informed policy and
        management, 153–4, 162–3
    inclusion criteria, 31
    iterative view of, 22
    and knowledge support, 13–15, 19–21
    and narrative synthesis, 103
    quality appraisal, 31–40
    questions to ask about, 181–4
    stages or elements in, 21–2
    and synthesis, 16, 17, 42–3
    writing up, 43

tabulation
    details of study designs, 121–2
    and narrative synthesis, 107
text-based data *see* qualitative research
    evidence
thematic analysis, 95, 96–7, 108
theoretical sampling, and grounded theory,
    77
third order interpretations, meta-
    ethnography of medicine-taking, 84–5
third order synthesis, in first generation
    literature reviews, 6

Thomas, J., 24–5, 109
Thomas, K., 179
time trends, 130, 131
translational synthesis methods, 45
  interpretive synthesis, 79–93
transparency
  in literature reviews, 5, 8
  in presentation of research, 150–1
  in systematic reviews, 19
tree plots, 130
triangulation, 179–80
  and narrative synthesis, 109
truth tables, and qualitative comparative
  analysis, 68–70
Turner, Stephen, 80
two communities model, of evidence-policy
  relationships, 158–62, 165, 168,
  170

validity assessment, 110
Van Maanen, J., 137, 151
visual displays of synthesis material, 121–26
vote-counting
  as a descriptive tool, 123–6
  and narrative synthesis, 107

Weber, Max, 72
Weight of Evidence, 109
Weiss, C.H., 155–6, 157, 158
White, C., 163
World Wide Web, 3, 4
writing up systematic reviews, 43
written reports, structure and format of,
  138–40

Yates, D., 52
Yin, R., 52, 53, 55, 78

DOING A LITERATURE REVIEW IN HEALTH AND SOCIAL CARE
A PRACTICAL GUIDE

Helen Aveyard

- Why do a literature review?
- What literature is relevant to my review?
- How do I appraise my findings?
- How do I present my literature review?

This book is a step-by-step guide to doing a literature review in health and social care. It is crucial reading for all those undertaking their undergraduate or postgraduate dissertation or any research module which involves a literature review. This student-friendly book:

- Simplifies the complex process of systematically reviewing published literature
- Provides a guide to searching, appraising and comparing literature to address a research question

Beginning with a discussion of the difference between a systematic and narrative review, you are then advised how to conduct a literature review, starting with defining the question, followed by strategies for searching the literature and emphasising the key elements that need to be considered when reviewing each kind of study. Throughout the book, there are practical tips on how to write up a literature review.

Doing a Literature Review is essential reading for all undergraduate students who are writing a literature based dissertation within the health and social care field, or as an introductory text for postgraduate study. It is also a useful text for those who are new to reviewing and appraising literature in the search for answers to questions that arise in practice.

Contents
Introduction – Why do a literature review? – What literature will be relevant to my review? – How do I develop a research question? – How do I search for literature? – How do I critically appraise the literature? – How do I synthesise my findings? – How do I discuss my findings and make recommendations? – How do I present my literature review? – Commonly asked questions – Glossary – References.

216pp
978–0–335–22261–2 (Paperback)   978–0–335–22262–9 (Hardback)

HANDBOOK OF HEALTH RESEARCH METHODS
INVESTIGATION, MEASUREMENT AND ANALYSIS

Ann Bowling and Shah Ebrahim (eds)

'an ideal set text'   Angela Scriven, Course Leader, Brunel University

- Which research method should I use to evaluate services?
- How do I design a questionnaire?
- How do I conduct a systematic review of research?

This handbook helps researchers to plan, carry out, and analyse health research, and evaluate the quality of research studies. The book takes a multidisciplinary approach to enable researchers from different disciplines to work side-by-side in the investigation of population health, the evaluation of health care, and in health care delivery.

Handbook of Health Research Methods is an essential tool for researchers and post-graduate students taking masters courses, or undertaking doctoral programmes, in health services evaluation, health sciences, health management, public health, nursing, sociology, socio-biology, medicine and epidemiology. However, the book also appeals to health professionals who wish to broaden their knowledge of research methods in order to make effective policy and practice decisions.

Contributors: Joy Adamson, Geraldine Barrett, Jane P. Biddulph, Ann Bowling, Sara Brookes, Jackie Brown, Simon Carter, Michel P. Coleman, Paul Cullinan, George Davey Smith, Paul Dieppe, Jenny Donovan, Craig Duncan, Shah Ebrahim, Vikki Entwistle, Clare Harries, Lesley Henderson, Kelvyn Jones, Olga Kostopoulou, Sarah J. Lewis, Richard Martin, Martin McKee, Graham Moon, Ellen Nolte, Alan O'Rourke, Ann Oakley, Tim Peters, Tina Ramkalawan, Caroline Sanders, Mary Shaw, Andrew Steptoe, Jonathan Sterne, Anne Stiggelbout, S.V. Subramanian, Kate Tilling, Liz Twigg, Suzanne Wait.

Contents

Section 1: Introduction – Introduction: research on health and health care – Describing and evaluating health systems – *Section 2: Multidisciplinary methods of investigation* – Evidence based health care: systematic reviews – Critical appraisal – Features and designs of randomised and non-randomised controlled trials and non-randomised experimental designs – Epidemiological study designs in health care research and evaluation – Finding and using secondary data on the health and health care of populations – Quantitative social science: The survey – Approaches to qualitative data collection in social science – Combined qualitative and quantitative designs – Design and analysis of social inter-vention studies in health research – Area-based studies and the evaluation of multilevel influences on health outcomes – Mathematical models in health care – Economic evalu-ation of health care – *Section 3: Multidisciplinary research measurement* – Psycho-logical approaches to measuring and modelling clinical decision making – Approaches to measuring patients' decision making – Techniques of questionnaire design – Measuring health outcomes from the patient's perspective – Genetics, health and population genetics research – Tools of psychosocial biology and health care research – *Section 4: Data analysis* – Key issues in the statistical analysis of quantitative data in research on health and health services – Key issues in the analysis of qualitative data on health services research – *Section 5: Essential issues to consider when conducting research* – Involving service users in health services research – Ethical and political issues in the conduct of research – Training for research – General glossary – General further reading – Index.

640pp   978–0–335–21460–0 (Paperback)   978–0–335–21461–7 (Hardback)

SUCCESSFUL QUALITATIVE HEALTH RESEARCH
A PRACTICAL INTRODUCTION

Emily Hansen

I like the way the author spends time on the background to and planning of qualitative research, rather than leaping straight into methods, which is what students tend to do! Descriptions and explanations of theoretical and practical aspects of qualitative work are combined well at a level that will engage students and professionals alike. The chapters on methods of qualitative data collection in particular are comprehensive with many helpful practical tips.

Catherine Perry, University of Chester, UK

I strongly recommend this book to all those looking to undertake ethical and rigorous qualitative research in the field of health and health care.

Jon Adams, University of Newcastle, Australia and University of Leeds, UK

A practical overview for health students and health professionals embarking on an applied research project using a qualitative approach.

Successful Qualitative Health Research offers a thorough introduction to the field, written in a clear and concise fashion. Emphasising the rigorous approach required in health research, it provides a step-by-step guide to designing a research project using qualitative methods, and to collecting, analysing and presenting different types of data.

Hansen provides essential insights into the ideas and arguments underpinning different qualitative methods, and highlights the links between theory and practice. She also explains the importance of choosing the most appropriate form of data analysis. Each chapter features real life examples from experienced researchers from a wide range of health fields. These examples show how researchers have overcome common problems and offer inspiration and guidance.

Applied qualitative research is increasingly being used to explore a range of issues in health, both on its own and as an adjunct to quantitative research. This book offers a clear, no-nonsense approach that will be invaluable to students and professionals in nursing, medicine, allied health and public health.

Contents
Preface – Acknowledgements – Qualitative research: An introduction – Planning your research – Research design and rigour – Observation and participant observation – Interviewing – Focus groups – Analysing qualitative data – Writing qualitative research – Glossary – References – Index.

240pp
978–0–335–22034–2 (Paperback)   978–0–335–22035–9 (Hardback)